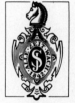

F. Wachsmann   G. Drexler

Graphs and Tables for Use in Radiology
Kurven und Tabellen für die Radiologie
Graphiques et Tables pour la Radiologie
Gráficas y Tablas para Radiología

With the collaboration of – Unter Mitarbeit von
Avec la collaboration de – Con la colaboración de

K. Bunzl   M. Busch   H. Czempiel   J. David   M. Gossrau
G. Grünauer   R. G. Jaeger   H. L. Keller   H. Oeser   W. Panzer
H. Paretzke   K. R. Trott   L. Widenmann

Second completely revised and enlarged edition
Zweite, völlig neu bearbeitete und erweiterte Auflage
Deuxième édition revisée et completée
Segunda edición totalmente revisada y aumentada

Springer-Verlag Berlin Heidelberg New York 1976

Professor Dr.-Ing. Felix Wachsmann

Dr.-Ing. Günter Drexler

Institut für Strahlenschutz
Gesellschaft für Strahlen- und Umweltforschung mbH,
8042 Neuherberg bei München

Titel der ersten Auflage: Kurven und Tabellen für die Strahlentherapie
© S. Hirzel Verlag, Stuttgart 1957

ISBN 3-540-07809-6 Springer-Verlag Berlin Heidelberg New York
ISBN 0-387-07809-6 Springer-Verlag New York Heidelberg Berlin

Library of Congress Cataloging in Publication Data. Wachsmann, Felix, 1904-. Graphs and tables for use in radiology = Kurven und Tabellen für die Radiologie. First ed. (c 1957) published under title: Kurven und Tabellen für die Strahlentherapie. Text in English, French, German, and Spanish. Bibliography: p. Includes index. 1. Radiology, Medical-Tables. I. Drexler, Günter, 1935-, joint author. II. Title. III. Title: Kurven und Tabellen für die Radiologie. R895.W3 1976 616.07'57'0212 76-14437

Druck: fotokop wilhelm weihert KG, Darmstadt
Bindearbeiten: Universitätsdruckerei H. Stürtz AG, Würzburg

The authors wish to thank:
Die Verfasser danken:
Les auteurs remercient:
Los autores agradecen a:

For valuable suggestions and for the translation of the texts into
English, French, and Spanish
Für wertvolle Anregungen und die Übersetzung der Texte ins Englische,
Französische und Spanische
Pour leurs précieuses suggestions et pour leurs traductions en ang-
lais, français et espagnol
Por sus valiosas sugestiones y la traducción de los textos al Inglés,
Francés y Espagnol

       M. Cohen, Montreal; Mrs. E. Lanzl, Chicago
       Mme A. Dutreix, Paris
       R.D. Perches, Mexico City; M.D. Reboiras, Madrid;

for the typing of the text, the drawings, and the photographic work,
für das Schreiben des Textes, das Zeichnen der Graphiken und die Er-
ledigung der Fotoarbeiten
pour la dactylographie du texte, les dessins, et le travail photogra-
phique,
por la escritura del texto, diagramas, y el trabajo de fotografiado,

       K. Semmelmann, I. Zink, I. Schellmann;

for making possible the work performed at the Gesellschaft für Strah-
len- und Umweltforschung mbH Munich, the scientific director
für die Ermöglichung der Arbeiten bei der Gesellschaft für Strahlen-
und Umweltforschung mbH München ihrem Wissenschaftlichen Geschäftsfüh-
rer,
pour avoir rendu possible le travail effectué au Gesellschaft für
Strahlen- und Umweltforschung mbH Munich, son directeur scientifique
por hacer posible le realización del trabajo en la Gesellschaft für
Strahlen- und Umweltforschung mbH Munich a su director scientifico

       R. Wittenzellner;

for the publication of the book, and for its responsiveness to our
wishes, the
für die Herausgabe und das verständnisvolle Eingehen auf unsere Wünsche dem
pour la publication et pour la compréhension de nos désirs
por la publicación, y comprensión de a nuestros deseos

       Springer-Verlag, Heidelberg

Foreword

The first edition of this book was published more than 15 years ago and created considerable interest among radiotherapists and medical physicists. The present new edition takes into consideration the latest scientific developments. It is a completely revised version and the information included has been considerably expanded. The presentation of the material in different languages and in the form of adjacent tables and diagrams is of particular value because it enables the reader to choose the presentation he prefers.

Whereas the data in the first edition were mainly related to radiotherapy, the new edition also includes information on nuclear medicine, X-ray diagnosis, radiation protection, and biomedical findings.

I hope that this book will be of value to a wide range of readers throughout the world and I am convinced that its use in daily work will contribute considerably to the badly needed improvement in the medical applications of ionizing radiation.

Professor Dr. W. Seelentag
Chief Medical Officer, Radiation Medicine
World Health Organization, Geneva

Vorwort

Die vor mehr als 15 Jahren erschienene 1. Auflage des vorliegenden Buches hatte bei Strahlentherapeuten und medizinischen Physikern großen Anklang gefunden. Die vorliegende Neuauflage wurde auf den neuesten Stand des Wissens gebracht, völlig neu bearbeitet und im Informationsgehalt wesentlich erweitert. Der besondere Wert des Buches liegt wiederum in der Mehrsprachigkeit und der parallelen Darstellung in Kurven und Tabellen, welche dem Leser erlauben, die ihm zusagende Darstellungsform zu benutzen.

Zu den in der 1. Auflage enthaltenen Kurven und Tabellen, die vorzugsweise auf die Strahlentherapie ausgerichtet waren, sind Abschnitte über Nuklearmedizin, Röntgendiagnostik und den Strahlenschutz hinzugekommen, sowie schließlich ein Abschnitt mit Zahlenangaben über allgemeine biologisch-medizinische Erkenntnisse.

Ich wünsche dem Buch eine gute Aufnahme in der ganzen Welt und bin davon überzeugt, daß sein Gebrauch in der täglichen Arbeit wesentlich zur dringend erforderlichen Verbesserung der medizinischen Strahlenanwendungen beitragen wird.

Professor Dr. W. Seelentag
Leiter der Abteilung Strahlenmedizin der
Weltgesundheitsorganisation, Genf

Avant - propos

Publiées pour la première fois il y a une quinzaine d'années, les "Courbes et Tables de Radiothérapie" ont suscité un très grand intérêt parmi les radiothérapeutes et les radiophysiciens. Depuis, les connaissances scientifiques ont beaucoup progressé, rendant nécessaire une mise à jour. Le présent volume contient donc une version complètement remaniée et complétée du texte précédent. La somme d'informations qui y figure est plus vaste que dans la première édition, et on retrouve dans la présente version un des grands avantages de la première, c'est-à-dire la présentation en plusieurs langues et des tables et courbes côte à côte, ce qui permet au lecteur de choisir la présentation qui lui convient le mieux.

Alors que la première édition était essentiellement consacrée à la radiothérapie, la nouvelle contient également des chapitres sur la médecine nucléaire, le radiodiagnostic et la radioprotection, ainsi que sur des données biomédicales générales.

J'espère que ce livre pourra être utile à une très large gamme d'utilisateurs dans le monde et je suis convaincu qu'il contribuera, dans la pratique quotidienne, à l'amélioration tant souhaitable des applications médicales des rayonnements ionisants.

Professeur Dr. W. Seelentag
Médecin Chef, Section de Médecine radiologique
Organisation Mondiale de la Santé, Genève

Prólogo

La primera edición del presente libro, aparecida hace más de 15 años, ha encontrado gran aceptación entre los radioterapeutas y físico-médicos. La presente edición ha sido puesta al día al nivel de los conocimientos actuales, totalmente refundida y sensiblemente aumentada en el contenido de sus materias. Por otro lado, el libro posee un valor especial al estar presentado en varios idiomas y ofrecer paralelamente representaciones gráficas y tablas que permiten al lector elegir la forma que más le convenga.

Además de las curvas y tablas de la 1ª edición, principalmente orientadas a la radioterapia, se incluye en esta, información sobre medicina nuclear, diagnóstico por rayos X y protección radioactiva, asi como una sección al final dedicada a datos numéricos sobre conocimientos generales de biomedicina.

Deseo que el libro alcance una buena acogida en todo el mundo y estoy convencido de que su manejo en el trabajo diario contribuirá apreciablemente a la urgente y necesaria mejora de las aplicaciones médicas de la radiación.

Profesor Dr. W. Seelentag
Director del Departamento de Medicina radiologica
de la Organización Mundial de la Salud, Ginebra

Table of contents

Detailed tables of contents can be found at the beginning of each section on the pages listed below:

Inhaltsverzeichnis

Die aufgegliederten Inhaltsverzeichnisse befinden sich am Anfang der einzelnen Abschnitte auf den nachstehend genannten Seiten:

Table des matières

Les tables des matières détaillées se trouvent au commencement de chaque chapitre sur les pages suivantes:

Tabla de materias

Las tablas de materias detalladas se encuentran en el comienzo de cada capítulo en las páginas que se indican:

Table of contents - Inhaltsverzeichnis
Table des matières - Tabla de materias

1.1 Editors' Comments

In this book, the numerical data needed by the radiologist and radiation physicist are given in the form of <u>graphs and tables:</u>

<u>Graphic representations</u> were chosen when it was important primarily to show the relationship between variables. Graphs have the additional advantages of providing information rapidly and of making available any desired intermediate values.

<u>Tables,</u> on the other hand, provide specific values with greater speed and reliability, and often with greater precision than graphs. For many topics in which not only a representation by curves, but also the easy availability of particular numbers was important, graphs and tables were placed side by side.

The <u>accuracy</u> of the tables was chosen to correspond to practical needs. We avoided the use of uncertain decimal places which would give the impression of pseudoaccuracy. In particular cases where it was impossible to give precise values, we used the designation "average or approximate values". If numbers cited in the literature were not in agreement, a critical selection of the most probable values according to our present knowledge was made. Special attention was paid to making the values given in the various graphs and tables compatible to facilitate comparison. <u>Uncertain values</u> were indicated in the graphs by dotted lines and <u>in the tables, by</u> parentheses.

<u>The material was chosen</u> in such a way that the data needed in daily practice are as complete as possible. Due to the limitations of the length of the book, however, this goal could not be attained perfectly. In addition, we included some material in which <u>general relationships</u> can be recognized qualitatively, and which may be of interest to those users of the graphs and tables who need information on related subjects.

The <u>literature</u> cited under the individual subjects is by no means complete. Instead, particularly those reports and textbooks were selected from which additional information can be obtained. Unfortunately it was impossible to have English-American, German, French, and Spanish literature represented equally.

The texts for the graphs and tables are given in four <u>languages.</u> The resulting space limitations forced us to use brief formulations; we hope that these are always clear. In exceptional cases, especially in some tables, only English, or Latin for medical terms, was used when this seemed possible without creating linguistic problems.

Some <u>difficulties</u> arose, for example, the marking of decimal fractions by periods or commas or, in the English text, the use of British or American spelling; we consistently used the British form. If we have not succeeded in satisfying all demands, we ask the reader's forbearance.

The Editors

1.1 Bemerkungen der Herausgeber

Das vom Radiologen und Strahlenphysiker benötigte Zahlenmaterial ist
im vorliegenden Buch in Kurven und Tabellen wiedergegeben:

Graphische Darstellungen wurden dort gewählt, wo es vor allem darauf
ankam, den Verlauf von Zusammenhängen zu zeigen. Diese bieten darüber
hinaus den Vorteil einer schnellen Information und daß aus ihnen be-
liebige Zwischenwerte abgelesen werden können.

Tabellen dagegen lassen Einzelwerte schneller, sicherer und oft ge-
nauer ablesen als Kurven. Bei vielen Themen, bei denen es sowohl auf
die Darstellung des Verlaufes als auch auf die bequeme Ablesbarkeit
von Einzelwerten ankam, wurden Kurven und Tabellen nebeneinander ge-
stellt.

Die Genauigkeit der angegebenen Werte ist so gewählt, daß sie prak-
tischen Bedürfnissen entspricht. Es wurde vermieden, durch Angabe
nicht gesicherter Dezimalstellen eine Pseudogenauigkeit vorzutäuschen.
Bei einzelnen Darstellungen, bei denen genaue Werte anzugeben unmög-
lich ist, wurde dies durch den Vermerk "Richtwerte" gekennzeichnet.
Wenn in der Literatur voneinander abweichende Werte genannt sind,
wurden die nach unserem heutigen Wissen wahrscheinlichsten kritisch
ausgewählt bzw. Mittelwerte gebildet. Es wurde besonders darauf ge-
achtet, daß die in den verschiedenen Kurven und Tabellen genannten
Werte miteinander vergleichbar sind. Unsichere Werte wurden in den
graphischen Darstellungen durch gestrichelte Linien und in den Tabellen dadurch gekennzeichnet, daß die Zahlenwerte in Klammern gesetzt
wurden.

Die Auswahl des Stoffes erfolgte so, daß die in der täglichen Praxis
benötigten Angaben möglichst vollständig aufgenommen wurden. Mit
Rücksicht auf den Umfang des Buches ließ sich dieses Ziel leider nicht
vollständig erreichen. Darüber hinaus wurden aber auch einige Darstellungen gebracht, die allgemeine Zusammenhänge qualitativ erkennen
lassen und für die Benutzer der Kurven und Tabellen von Interesse sein
mögen, um sich über Randgebiete zu informieren.

Die bei den einzelnen Themen angegebene Literatur ist keineswegs vollständig! Es wurden vielmehr bevorzugt nur solche Arbeiten und Lehr-
bücher zitiert, aus denen weitere Informationen entnommen werden können. Dabei konnte die deutsche, englisch-amerikanische, französische
und spanische Literatur leider nicht gleichmäßig berücksichtigt werden.

Die Kurven und Tabellen sind grundsätzlich viersprachig beschriftet.
Der hierdurch bedingte Platzbedarf hat zu knappen Formulierungen ge-
zwungen, die hoffentlich immer verständlich sind. Nur in Ausnahmefäl-
len, d.h. besonders in einigen Tabellen, wurde dort, wo dies möglich
erschien, ohne sprachliche Schwierigkeiten aufkommen zu lassen, nur
englisch bzw. bei medizinischen Ausdrücken lateinisch beschriftet.

Schwierigkeiten ergaben sich auch z.B. bezüglich der Kennzeichnung
von Dezimalbrüchen durch Punkt oder Komma oder im Englischen bezüglich der englischen oder amerikanischen Schreibweise; wir wählten ein-
heitlich die englische. Wenn wir dabei nicht alle Wünsche erfüllt haben, bitten wir um Nachsicht.

Die Verfasser

1.1 Commentaires des editeurs

Dans ce livre, les valeurs numériques nécessaires aux radiologistes et aux radiophysiciens sont données sous la forme de <u>graphiques et de tables</u>:

La <u>représentation graphique</u> a été choisie chaque fois qu'il a paru surtout important de montrer les relations entre variables. Les graphiques présentent en outre l'avantage de fournir rapidement les informations et de faciliter la détermination pour des valeurs intermédiaires des variables.

<u>Les tables</u>, d'autre part, fournissent des valeurs en des points spécifiques, plus rapidement, de façon plus fiable et souvent avec une plus grande précision que les graphiques. Dans de nombreux cas, pour lesquels la représentation graphique, mais également la disponibilité de valeurs numériques est importante, les graphiques et les tables ont été placés l'un à côté de l'autre.

La <u>précision</u> des valeurs a été choisie en fonction des besoins pratiques. Nous avons évité d'utiliser des décimales qui donneraient une impression de pseudoprécision. Dans les cas particuliers où il est impossible de donner des valeurs précises, nous avons utilisé l'expression "valeurs moyennes" ou "valeurs approchées". Lorsque les valeurs citées dans la littérature ne sont pas en accord, une sélection critique des valeurs les plus probables suivant l'état actuel de nos connaissances, a été effectuée. On s'est assuré tout spécialement de la compatibilité des valeurs données dans les différents tableaux et graphiques afin de faciliter les comparaisons. <u>Les valeurs qui ne sont pas très sûres</u> sont indiquées dans les graphiques par des lignes pointillées et dans les tables par des parenthèses.

<u>Le choix</u> a été fait de façon à ce que les données nécessaires dans la pratique quotidienne soient aussi complètes que possible. Cependant, du fait de la limite imposée à la taille de ce livre, ce but n'a pu être atteint parfaitement. En outre, nous avons ajouté quelques données montrant des <u>relations générales</u> qualitatives et pouvant être utiles aux lecteurs qui recherchent des informations sur des sujets en rapport avec ceux traités dans les tables et les graphiques.

<u>Les références bibliographiques</u> citées ne sont en aucune façon complètes. Au contraire on a choisi seulement les rapports et les livres dans lesquels des informations supplémentaires pouvaient être trouvées. Malheureusement il a été impossible de représenter également les littératures française, anglaise, américaine, allemande et espagnole.

Les textes accompagnant les graphiques et les tables sont donnés en <u>quatre langues</u>. En conséquence, l'espace a été très limité et nous avons été obligés d'utiliser des expressions très simples. Dans quelques cas exceptionnels, spécialement dans certaines tables, seul l'Anglais ou le Latin a été utilisé. Nous espérons qu'elles sont néanmoins toujours claires. Nous avons rencontré quelques <u>difficultés</u>: par exemple, la séparation des fractions décimales par des points ou des virgules, ou encore, le choix entre les orthographes britanniques ou américaines; nous avons toujours choisi la forme britannique. Nous demandons l'indulgence du lecteur si nous n'avons pas réussi à satisfaire à toutes des demandes.

Les Editeurs

1.1 Notas de los editores

El presente libro ofrece en curvas y tablas, los datos numéricos que
necesitan el radiólogo y el radio-físico.

Las representeciones gráficas se eligieron cuando se consideró apropiado poner de manifiesto la dependencia continua entre variables.
Estas ofrecen, además de la ventaja de una rápida información, la
posibilidad de lectura de valores intermedios.

Las tablas, por el contrario, permiten leer valores particulares de
forma más rápida, segura y exacta que en las curvas. En muchos temas,
en los cuales hubo que atender tanto a la representación gráfica como
a la lectura cómoda de una magnitud, se ofrecen las curvas y tablas
unas al lado de las otras.

La exactitud de los valores se ha elegido de forma que corresponda a
las necesidades prácticas. Se ha querido evitar el hacer creer en
una pseudoexactitud dando cifras decimales que no son seguras. En casos particulares, en los que es imposible dar valores exactos, se indicaron estos mediante la notación "valores estimativos". En el caso
de valores que se encuentran en la literatura y se desvian entre si,
se eligieron con criterio crítico los más probables, de acuerdo con
nuestros conocimientos actuales, o se estimaron los valores medios.
Se ha puesto especial cuidado en que los valores indicados en diferentes curvas y tablas sean comparables entre si. Los valores inseguros se indicaron en la representaciones gráficas mediante líneas ar-
ticuladas y en las tablas poniendolos entre paréntesis.

En la elección de la temática se tuvo en cuenta que estuvieran reco-
gidos de forma lo más completa posible los datos necesarios en la
práctica diaria. Este fin, por desgracia, no se ha podido alcanzar
totalmente en consideración a la extensión del libro. Además se in-
cluyen algunas gráficas en las que se recogen relaciones generales
cualitativas y que son de interés para el manejo de las curvas y
tablas, para informarse sobre cuestiones adicionales.

La literatura indicada para cada tema particular no es de ninguna
forma exhaustiva! Se prefirió mucho antes citar solamente aquellos
trabajos y tratados, que puedan proporcionar informaciones más am-
plias.

Las curvas y tablas llevan una leyenda en cuatro idiomas; por ello,
las disponibilidades de espacio nos han obligado a formulaciones
abreviadas que esperamos resulten siempre comprensivas. Unicamente
en casos escepcionales, concretamente en algunas tablas, se escribió
solo inglés, o latin en expresiones médicas, pero unicamente en
aquellos casos en que ha sido posible sin crear dificultades de com-
prensibilidad.

Dificultades han surgido también por ejemplo en lo referente a la
utilización del punto o la coma en los números decimales o en las
formas de expresión inglesas o americanas; nosotros hemos elegido
siempre las inglesas. Si con ello no hemos satisfecho todas las exi-
gencias, rogamos indulgencia para

los autores

15

1.2 Abbreviations and symbols

1.2   Decimal fraction: "1 unit, 2 tenths"; instead of the notation used in Germany and France: 1,2

x   multiplication sign (e.g., "2 x 3 = 6"); in equations also ·
(e.g., "2·3 = 6")

=   equals

∿   similar to (approximately equal)

≈   approximately (nearly or practically equal)
(the two penultimate symbols, respectively≋ placed after "V"
the abbreviation for the unit of voltage, e.g., "kV=, kV∿, or

≋   kV≋", mean direct-current voltage, alternating-current voltage, or threephase alternating current)

>   greater than ... (e.g., "8>5")

<   less than ... (e.g., "5<8")

decimal fractions and multiples: a, f, p, n, μ, m, c, k, M,
G, T, P, E (10^{-18}...10^{18}); for details, see page 41

ℓ   liter (unit of volume)

m   meter (SI unit of length)

g   gram (unit of mass; SI unit kg)

s   second (SI unit of time)

min   minute (unit of time)

h   hour (hora - unit of time)

d   day (dies - unit of time)

a   year (annum - unit of time)

T   time (tempus - general)

$T_{1/2}$ half-life (time in which half of a radioactive substance
decays); also HL

τ   lifetime (= time in which a radioactive substance has decayed
to 1/e, i.e. to about 37% of the initial value)

A   ampere (SI unit of electrical current)

V   volt (unit of electric potential)

C   coulomb (SI unit of electric charge)

W   watt (SI unit of power)

J   joule (SI unit of energy)

mAs   milliampere-second (quantity used for radiographic exposures)

R   röntgen (unit of exposure)

rad   rad (radiation absorbed dose = unit of absorbed dose)

Gy   gray (SI unit of absorbed dose)

rem   rem (radiation equivalent man = equivalent dose)

Ci   curie (unit of radioactivity, = $3.71 \cdot 10^{10}$ decays/s)

Bq   becquerel (SI unit of radioactivity; = 1 decay/s)

RBE   relative biologic effectiveness

q   quality factor (= RBE for radiation protection, for values
see p.44)

e	1. elementary electric charge (see page 40) and 2. basis of the natural logarithm (e = 2.718282)
eV	electron volt (unit of energy, 1 J = $6.2435 \cdot 10^{18}$ eV)
LET	linear energy transfer (energy discharged by a particle during its passage through matter per unit path length)
°C	degree centigrad (unit of temperature referred to the freezing point of water)
°F	degrees Fahrenheit (unit of temperature referred to -32°C)
K	kelvin (formerly degrees Kelvin) unit of temperature referred to the absolute zero point -273°C
α	alpha (symbol for alpha particles or alpha radiation)
β	beta (symbol for beta particles or beta radiation)
γ	gamma (symbol for gamma particles or gamma radiation)
n	neutron (particles or radiation)
p	proton (particles or radiation)
e^-, e^+	electron resp. positron (particles or radiation)
d	deuteron (particles or radiation)
Γ	gamma (specific gamma-ray constant, $\frac{R \cdot m^2}{h \cdot Ci}$, see page 150)
η	eta (symbol for degree of effectiveness)
ρ	rho (symbol for the density of a substance)
λ	lambda (symbol for the wavelength of radiation)
FSD	focus-skin (surface)-distance
SD	source distance
SSD	source-skin-(surface)-distance
HVL	half-value layer (measure of the energy of a radiation)
HVD	half-value depth in tissue
MPC	maximum permissible concentration
D	dose (general)
$\overline{D}$	(time) average of the dose ($\overline{X}$ general = time average of a quantity)
$\dot{D}$	dose rate ($\dot{X}$ general = time-related quantity)
D_0	dose which kills 1 - 1/e (= 63%) of irradiated individuals
LD_{50}	lethal dose 50, i.e., dose by which 50% of irradiated individuals are killed
$^3_1 H$	hydrogen (or other chemical elements, as on page 24 and 27) with the atomic number 1 written as subscript before the symbol and the mass number 3 as superscript before the symbol
SI	International System of Units
ICRU	International Commission on Radiation Units and Measurements
ICRP	International Commission on Radiological Protection
ISO	International Standard Organisation
DIN	German Standard Institute (Deutsches Institut für Normung)

1.2 Abkürzungen und Formelzeichen

1.2   Dezimalbruch: 1 Ganzes, 2 Zehntel (anstelle der in der deut-
        schen und französischen benutzen Schreibweise: 1,2)

x   Zeichen für Multiplikation (z.B. 2 x 3 = 6); in Formeln auch: ·
        (z.B. 2·3 = 6)

=   gleich

∿   ähnlich (ungefähr gleich)

≈   angenähert (nahezu oder praktisch) gleich
        (diese drei Symbole hinter dem Kurzzeichen für die Einheit der
        Spannung V (z.B. kV=, kV∿ oder kV≈) bedeuten Gleichspannung,
        Wechselspannung oder Drehstrom)

>   größer als ... (z.B. 8>5)
<   kleiner als ... (z.B. 5<8)

        Dezimale Brüche und Vielfache a, f, p, n, µ, m, c, k, M, G, T,
        P, E ($10^{-18}...10^{18}$), siehe Seite 41

ℓ   Liter (Einheit des Volumens)

m   Meter (SI-Längeneinheit)

g   Gramm (Masseneinheit; SI-Einheit kg)

s   Sekunde (SI-Zeiteinheit)

min   Minute (Zeiteinheit)

h   Stunde (hora - Zeiteinheit)

d   Tag (dies - Zeiteinheit)

a   Jahr (annum - Zeiteinheit)

T   Zeit (tempus - allgemein)

$T_{1/2}$ Halbwertzeit (Zeit, in der die Hälfte eines radioaktiven Stof-
        fes zerfallen ist) auch HWZ

τ   mittlere Lebensdauer (= Zeit, in der ein radioaktiver Stoff
        auf 1/e, d.h. rund 37 % des Ausganswertes, zerfallen ist)

A   Ampere (SI-Einheit der elektrischen Stromstärke)

V   Volt (Einheit der elektrischen Spannung)

W   Watt (SI-Einheit der Leistung)

J   Joule (SI-Einheit der Energie)

mAs   Milli-Ampere-Sekunden Produkt (zur Kennzeichnung der für die
        Belichtung von Röntgenaufnahmen benutzten Größe)

R   Röntgen (Einheit der Ionendosis)

rad   Rad (radiation absorbed dose - Einheit der Energiedosis; in
        Deutschland Abkürzung auch rd)

Gy   Gray (Si-Einheit der Energiedosis)

rem   rem (radiation equivalent man - Äquivalentdosis)

Ci   Curie (Einheit der Radioaktivität = $3,71·10^{10}$ Zerfälle/s)

Bq   Becquerel (SI-Einheit der Radioaktivität in Zerfällen/s)

RBW   Relative Biologische Wirksamkeit (englisch RBE)

q   Qualitätsfaktor (= RBW für Strahlenschutzzwecke abgerundet
        festgelegte Werte   siehe Seite 44)

C	Coulomb (SI-Einheit der elektrischen Ladung)
e	1. elektrische Elementarladung (siehe Seite 40) und 2. Basis des natürlichen Logarithmensystems (e = 2,718282)
eV	Elektronenvolt (Einheit der Energie, 1 J = 6,2435·10^{18} eV)
LET	Linear Energy Transfer (Energie, die ein Teilchen beim Durchgang durch Materie je Weglänge abgibt), deutsch auch LEÜ
°C	Grad Celsius (auf den Gefrierpunkt des Wassers bezogene Einheit der Temperatur)
°F	Grad Fahrenheit (auf -32°C bezogene Einheit der Temperatur, siehe Seite 42)
K	Kelvin (auf den absoluten Nullpunkt -273°C bezogene SI-Einheit der Temperatur °C, °F und K, siehe Seite 42)
α	Alpha (Symbol für Alpha-Teilchen oder Alpha-Strahlung)
β	Beta (Symbol für Beta-Teilchen oder Beta-Strahlung)
γ	Gamma (Symbol für Gamma-Quanten oder Gamma-Strahlung)
e⁻,e⁺	Elektron bzw. Positron (Teilchen oder Strahlung)
p	Proton (Teilchen oder Strahlung)
d	Deuteron (Teilchen oder Strahlung)
n	Neutron (Teilchen oder Strahlung)
Γ	Gamma (spezifische Gamma-Strahlenkonstante in $\frac{R \cdot m^2}{h \cdot Ci}$, s.Seite 150)
η	Eta (Symbol für Wirkungsgrad)
ρ	Rho (Symbol für die Dichte eines Stoffes)
λ	Lamda (Symbol für die Wellenlänge einer Strahlung)
FA	Fokusabstand (englisch FD, SD) bzw. QA = Quellenabstand
FHA	Fokus-Haut-Abstand (englisch FSD)
HWSD	Halbwertschichtdicke (Maß für die Härte einer Strahlung; englisch HVL)
GHWT	Gewebehalbwerttiefe (englisch HVD)
MZK	maximal zulässige Konzentration (englisch MPC)
D	Dosis (allgemein)
$\overline{D}$	(zeitlicher) Mittelwert der Dosis ($\overline{X}$ allgemein zeitlicher Mittelwert)
$\dot{D}$	Dosisleistung ($\dot{X}$ allgemein auf die Zeit bezogene Größe)
D_0	Dosis, die 1 - 1/e (= 63%) der bestrahlten Individuen abtötet
LD_{50}	Letal Dosis 50, d.h. Dosis, durch die 50 % der bestrahlten Individuen abgetötet werden
^3_1H	Wasserstoff (bzw. andere chemische Elemente)mit der Ordnungszahl 1 vor dem Symbol tiefgestellt und der Massenzahl 3 vor dem Symbol hochgestellt, siehe Seite 24 und 27
SI	Internationales Einheitensystem
ICRU	International Commission on Radiation Units and Measurements
ICRP	International Commission on Radiological Protection
ISO	International Standard Organisation
DIN	Deutsches Institut für Normung

1.2 Abréviations et symboles

1.2   fraction décimale: 1 unité, 2 dixièmes (au lieu de la notation française ou allemande 1,2)

x   signe de multiplication (par ex. 2 x 3 = 6); en formule aussi· (par ex. 2·3 = 6)

=   égale

∿   semblable à (à peu près égal)

≈   valeur approchée (presque égal ou pratiquement égal) (les deux derniers symboles, ainsi que le symbole ≋, placés après "V" l'abréviation pour l'unité de tension (par ex. kV=,

≋   kV∿, ou kV≋), signifient tension constante, tension alternative ou tension alternative triphasée)

>   plus grand que... (par ex. 8>5)

<   plus petit que... (par ex. 5<8)

   multiples et sous-multiples a, f, p, n, µ, m, c, k, M, G, T, P, E $(10^{-18}...10^{18})$ pour plus de détails, voir page 41

ℓ   litre (unité de volume)

m   mètre (unité SI de longueur)

g   gramme (unité de masse; SI unité kg)

s   seconde (unité SI de temps)

min   minute (unité de temps)

h   heure (unité de temps)

d   jour (dies - unité de temps)

a   année (annum - unité de temps)

T   temps (tempus - en général)

$T_{1/2}$ période demi vie, PDV (temps au bout duquel la moitié des atomes radioactifs se sont désintégrés)

τ   durée de vie (= temps au bout duquel une substance radioactiv a décru à 1/e = ∿37% de la valeur initiale)

A   Ampère (unité SI de courant électrique)

V   Volt (unité de potentiel électrique)

C   Coulomb (unité SI de charge électrique)

W   Watt (unité SI de puissance)

J   Joule (unité SI d'énergie)

mAs   milliampère seconde (quantité utilisée pour les radiographies)

R   röntgen (unité d'exposition)

rad   rad (radiation absorbed dose = unité de dose absorbée)

rem   rem (radiation equivalent man = dose équivalente)

Gy   gray (unité SI de dose absorbée)

Ci   Curie (ancienne unité de radioactivité = $3.71·10^{10}$ désintégrations/s)

Bq   Becquerel (unité SI de radioactivité = 1 désintégration/s)

EBR   efficacité biologique relative (anglais: RBE)

q	facteur de qualité (= EBR dans le domaine de la radioprotection; pour les valeurs approchées admises, voir page 44)
e	1. charge électrique élémentaire (voir page 40) et 2. base des logarithmes naturels (e = 2.718282)
eV	electron-volt (unité d'énergie. $1 J = 6.2435 \cdot 10^{18}$ eV)
TEL	transfert d'énergie linéique (anglais LET)
°C	degré centigrade (unité de température)
°F	degrés Fahrenheit (unité de température rapportée à -32°C)
K	Kelvin (auparavant degrés Kelvin) unité de température rapportée au zéro absolu (-273°C); °C, °F et K voir page 42
α	alpha (symbole pour particules ou rayonnement α)
β	beta (symbole pour particules ou rayonnement β)
γ	gamma (symbole pour particules ou rayonnement γ)
n	neutron (symbole pour particules ou rayonnement)
p	proton (symbole pour particules ou rayonnement)
d	deuteron (symbole pour particules ou rayonnement)
e^-, e^+	symboles pour les electrons et les positrons
Γ	gamma (constante de débit d'exposition; voir page 150)
η	eta (symbole pour le degré d'efficacité)
ρ	rho (symbole pour la densité d'une substance)
λ	lambda (symbole pour la longueur d'onde d'un rayonnement)
DFP	distance foyer-peau resp. DS distance de la source
CDA	couche de demi-atténuation (mesure de la qualité d'un rayonnement)
PDA	profondeur demi absorption tissulaire
CMA	concentration maximale admissible
D	dose (en général)
$\bar{D}$	dose moyenne (par rapport au temps) (en général $\bar{X}$ = moyenne d'une quantité X par rapport au temps)
$\dot{D}$	débit de dose (en général $\dot{X}$ = quantité X rapportée à l'unité de temps)
D_0	dose tuant $1 - 1/e$ (= 63%) d'individus irradiés
DL_{50}	dose létale 50, c'est-à-dire dose tuant 50% des individus irradiés
^3_1H	hydrogène (ou autre élément chimique décrit page 24) le nombre atomique 1 est écrit en bas et en avant du symbole et le nombre de masse 3 est écrit en haut en avant du symbole
SI	système international d'unites
ICRU	Commission internationale sur les unités radiologique (CIUR)
ICRP	Commission internationale sur la protection contre les radiations (CIPR)
ISO	Organisation internationale de normalisation
DIN	Institut allemand de normalisation (Deutsches Institut für Normung)

1.2 Abreviaturas y símbolos

1.2 número decimal: 1 unidad, 2 decena (en lugar de la forma usual de escritura alemana y francesa: 1,2)

x   símbolo de multiplicación (p. ej. 2 x 3 = 6); en las fórmulas también: · (p. ej. 2·3 = 6)

=   igual a

∿   semejante (aproximadamente igual a)

≈   muy cerca de (casi o practicamente) igual; (estos tres símbolos después de las unidades de tensión V (p. ej. kV=, kV∿ o kV≋) indican corriente continua, alterna o trifásica respectivamente)

>   mayor que ... (p. ej. 8>5)

<   menor que ... (p. ej. 5<8)

     números decimales y exponenciales a, f, p, n, µ, m, c, k, M, G, T, P, E ($10^{-18} \ldots 10^{18}$), vease página 41

ℓ   litro (unidad de volumen)

m   metro (unidad de longitud en el SI)

g   gramo (unidad de masa; unidad en el SI kg)

s   segundo (unidad de tiempo en el SI)

min   minuto (unidad de tiempo)

h   hora (unidad de tiempo)

d   día (unidad de tiempo)

a   año (unidad de tiempo)

T   tiempo (en general)

$T_{1/2}$ período de vida media (tiempo en el cual se disgrega la mitad de una sustancia radiactiva) también PVM

τ   vida media (= tiempo en el cual una sustancia radiactiva se disgrega hasta $1/_e$, de su valor inicial)

A   amperio (unidad de intensidad de corriente eléctrica en el SI)

V   voltio (unidad tensión eléctrica)

W   watio (unidad de potencia en el SI)

J   julio (unidad de energía en el SI)

mAs   producto de miliamperios por segundo (para denominar la magnitud utilizada en la impresión de radiografias)

R   röntgen (unidad de dosis iónica o exposición)

rad   Rad (dosis absorbida - unidad de dosis de energía)

Gy   Gray (unidad de dosis de energía en el SI)

rem   rem (radiación equivalente en el hombre - dosis equivalente)

Ci   Curie (unidad de radioactividad = $3,71 \cdot 10^{10}$ desintegraciones/s)

Bq   Becquerel (unidad de radioactividad del SI en desintegraciones/s)

EBR   efectividad biológica relativa (en inglés RBE)

q   factor de calidad (= EBR valores fijos redondeados para el radioprotección, vease página 44)

C   Coulomb (unidad de carga eléctrica en el SI)

e	1. carga eléctrica elemental (vease pág. 40) y 2. base del sistema de logaritmos natural (e = 2,718282)
eV	electrónvoltio (unidad de energía, 1 J = $6,2435 \cdot 10^{18}$ eV)
TLE	transmisión lineal de energía (energía que cede una partícula al pasar a través de un determinada porción de materia; inglés RBE)
°C	grado Celsius (unidad de temperatura referida al punto de congelación del agua)
°F	grado Fahrenheit (unidad de temperatura referida a -32 °C, vease pág. 42)
K	Kelvin (unidad de temperatura en el SI referida al punto del cero absoluto -273 °C, °C, °F y K vease pág. 42)
α	alfa (símbolo para las partículas o rayos alfa)
β	beta (símbolo para las partículas o rayos beta)
γ	gamma (símbolo para los cuantos o rayos gamma)
e^-,e^+	electrón o positrón (partículas o radiación)
p	protón (partículas o radiación)
d	deuterón (partículas o radiación)
n	neutrón (partículas o radiación)
Γ	gamma (constante de radiación gamma específica en $\frac{R \cdot m^2}{h \cdot Ci}$, v.p.150)
η	eta (símbolo del grado de eficacia)
ρ	ro (símbolo de la densidad de una sustancia)
λ	lambda (símbolo de la longitud de onda de una radiación)
DF	distancia focal o distancia fuente (inglés FD)
DFP	distancia foco- o sea fuente-piel (inglés FSD o sea SSD)
CHR	capa hemirreductora (medida de la dureza de una radiación, inglés HVL)
PHR	Profundidad hemi-reductora (tejido)
CMP	concentración máxima permisible (inglés MPC)
D	dosis (en general)
$\bar{D}$	valor medio de la dosis (temporal) ($\bar{X}$ valor medio temporal en general)
$\dot{D}$	intensidad de la dosis (X en general magnitud referida al tiempo)
D_o	dosis, el 1 - 1/e (= 63 %) de individuos radiados muertos
LD	dosis letal 50, es decir, la dosis mediante la cual se morirían el 50 % de los individuos irradiados
^3_1H	hidrógeno (u otro elemento químico) con el número atómico 1 como subíndice antes del símbolo y número másico 3 como super-indice antes del símbolo, vease páginas 24 y 27
SI	Sistema de Unidades Internacional
ICRP	Comisión Internacional de Radioprotección
ICRU	Comisión Internacional de Unidades de Radiación
ISO	Organización Internacional de Normalización
DIN	Instituto Alemán de Normalización

Periodic chart of the elements - Periodensystem der Elemente -

	I	II	III	IV	V
1	$^{1}_{1}H$ Hydrogen Wasserstoff Hydrogène Hidrógeno				
2	$^{7}_{3}Li$ Lithium Lithium Lithium Litio	$^{9}_{4}Be$ Beryllium Beryllium Béryllium Berilio	$^{11}_{5}B$ Boron Bor Bore Boro	$^{12}_{6}C$ Carbon Kohlenstoff Carbone Carbono	$^{14}_{7}N$ Nitrogen Stickstoff Azote Nitrógeno
3	$^{23}_{11}Na$ Sodium Natrium Sodium Sodio	$^{24}_{12}Mg$ Magnesium Magnesium Magnésium Magnesio	$^{27}_{13}Al$ Aluminium Aluminium Aluminium Aluminio	$^{28}_{14}Si$ Silicon Silizium Silicium Silicio	$^{31}_{15}P$ Phosphorus Phosphor Phosphore Fósforo
4	$^{39}_{19}K$ β Potassium Kalium Potassium Potasio	$^{40}_{20}Ca$ Calcium Kalzium Calcium Calcio	$^{45}_{21}Sc$ Scandium Skandium Scandium Escandio	$^{48}_{22}Ti$ Titanium Titan Titane Titanio	$^{51}_{23}V$ Vanadium Vanadium Vanadium Vanadio
	$^{63}_{29}Cu$ Copper Kupfer Cuivre Cobre	$^{64}_{30}Zn$ Zinc Zink Zinc Cinc	$^{69}_{31}Ga$ Gallium Gallium Gallium Galio	$^{74}_{32}Ge$ Germanium Germanium Germanium Germanio	$^{75}_{33}As$ Arsenic Arsen Arsenic Arsénico
5	$^{85}_{37}Rb$ β Rubidium Rubidium Rubidium Rubidio	$^{88}_{38}Sr$ Strontium Strontium Strontium Estroncio	$^{89}_{39}Y$ Yttrium Yttrium Yttrium Itrio	$^{90}_{40}Zr$ Zirconium Zirkon Zirconium Circonio	$^{93}_{41}Nb$ Niobium Niob Niobium Niobio
	$^{107}_{47}Ag$ Silver Silber Argent Plata	$^{114}_{48}Cd$ Cadmium Kadmium Cadmium Cadmium	$^{115}_{49}In$ β Indium Indium Indium Indio	$^{120}_{50}Sn$ Tin Zinn Étain Estano	$^{121}_{51}Sb$ Antimony Antimon Antimoine Antimonio
6	$^{133}_{55}Cs$ Cesium Zäsium Césium Cesio	$^{138}_{56}Ba$ Barium Barium Barium Bario	57-71 Rare earths Seltene Erden Terres rares Tierras raras	$^{180}_{72}Hf$ Hafnium Hafnium Hafnium Hafnio	$^{181}_{73}Ta$ Tantalum Tantal Tantale Tántalo
	$^{197}_{79}Au$ Gold Gold Or Oro	$^{202}_{80}Hg$ Mercury Quecksilber Mercure Mercurio	$^{205}_{81}Tl$ Thallium Thallium Thallium Talio	$^{208}_{82}Pb$ Lead Blei Plomb Plomo	$^{209}_{83}Bi$ Bismuth Wismut Bismuth Bismuto
7	$^{223}_{87}Fr$ (α) Francium Francium Francium Francio	$^{226}_{88}Ra$ α Radium Radium Radium Radio	$^{227}_{89}Ac$ β Actinium Aktinium Actinium Actinio	$^{232}_{90}Th$ α Thorium Thorium Thorium Torio	$^{231}_{91}Pa$ α Protactinium Protaktinium Protactinium Protactinio

Système périodique des éléments - Tabla periódica de los elementos

VI	VII	VIII			O
					$^{4}_{2}$He Helium Helium Hélium Helio
$^{16}_{8}$O Oxygen Sauerstoff Oxygène Oxígeno	$^{19}_{9}$F Fluorine Fluor Fluor Flúor				$^{20}_{10}$Ne Neon Neon Néon Neón
$^{32}_{16}$S Sulphur Schwefel Soufre Azufre	$^{35}_{17}$Cl Chlorine Chlor Chlore Cloro				$^{40}_{18}$Ar Argon Argon Argon Argón
$^{52}_{24}$Cr Chromium Chrom Chrome Cromo	$^{55}_{25}$Mn Manganese Mangan Manganèse Manganeso	$^{56}_{26}$Fe Iron Eisen Fer Hierro	$^{59}_{27}$Co Cobalt Kobalt Cobalt Cobalto	$^{58}_{28}$Ni Nickel Nickel Nickel Níquel	
$^{80}_{34}$Se Selenium Selen Sélénium Selenio	$^{79}_{35}$Br Bromine Brom Brome Bromo				$^{84}_{36}$Kr Krypton Krypton Krypton Criptón
$^{98}_{42}$Mo Molybdenum Molybdän Molybdène Molibdeno	$^{99}_{43}$Tc(β) Technetium Technetium Technécium Tecnecio	$^{102}_{44}$Ru Ruthenium Ruthenium Ruthénium Rutenio	$^{103}_{45}$Rh Rhodium Rhodium Rhodium Rodio	$^{106}_{46}$Pd Palladium Palladium Palladium Paladio	
$^{130}_{52}$Te Tellurium Tellur Tellurium Teluro	$^{127}_{53}$I/$^{127}_{53}$J Iodine Jod Iode Iodo				$^{132}_{54}$X Xenon Xenon Xénon Xenón
$^{184}_{74}$W Wolfram Wolfram Tungstène Wolframò	$^{187}_{75}$Re β Rhenium Rhenium Rhénium Renio	$^{192}_{76}$Is Osmium Osmium Osmium Osmio	$^{193}_{77}$Ir Iridium Iridium Iridium Iridio	$^{195}_{78}$Pt Platinum Platin Platine Platino	
$^{210}_{84}$Po α Polonium Polonium Polonium Polonio	$^{211}_{85}$At(α) Astatine Astatin Astate Astatio				$^{222}_{86}$Rn α Radon Radon Radon Radón
$^{238}_{92}$U α Uranium Uran Uranium Uranio	93... Transuranic elements Transurane Transuraniens Transurànicos				

Rare earths (57 - 71) Seltene Erden Terres rares Tierras raras	$^{139}_{57}$La γ Lanthanum Lanthan Lanthane Lantano	$^{140}_{58}$Ce Cerium Zer Cérium Cerio	$^{141}_{59}$Pr Praseodymium Praseodym Praséodyme Praseodimio	$^{144}_{60}$Nd Neodymium Neodym Néodymium Neodimio
	$^{147}_{61}$Pm(β) Promethium Prometheum Prométhéum Promedio	$^{152}_{62}$Sm α Samarium Samarium Samarium Samario	$^{153}_{63}$Eu Europium Europium Europium Europio	$^{158}_{64}$Gd Gadolinium Gadolinium Gadolinium Gadolinio
	$^{159}_{65}$Tb Terbium Terbium Terbium Terbio	$^{164}_{66}$Dy Dysprosium Dysprosium Dysprosium Disprosio	$^{165}_{67}$Ho Holmium Holmium Holmium Holmio	$^{166}_{68}$Er Erbium Erbium Erbium Erbio
	$^{169}_{69}$Tm Thulium Thulium Thulium Tulio	$^{174}_{70}$Yb Ytterbium Ytterbium Ytterbium Iterbio	$^{175}_{71}$Cp β Lutecium Lutetium Lutécium Lutecio	

Transuranic elements (93 ...) Transurane Transuraniens Transurânicos	$^{237}_{93}$Np(β) Neptunium Neptunio	$^{239}_{94}$Pu(α) Plutonium Plutonio	$^{241}_{95}$Am(α) Americium Americo
	$_{96}$Cm(α) Curium Curio	$_{97}$Bk(α) Berkelium Bercelio	$_{98}$Cf(α) Californium Californio
	$_{99}$Es Einsteinium Einsteinio	$_{100}$Fm Fermium Fermio	$_{101}$Md Mendelevium Mendelevio
	$_{102}$No Nobelium Nobelio	$_{103}$Lr Lawrencium Lawrencio	$_{104}$Ku Kurchatovium Kurchatovio
	$_{105}$Ha Hahnium	$_{106}$	

Note - Bemerkung - Remarque - Nota:

The index left of each symbol on the lower bottom is the atomic number and that on the upper the mass number of the most frequent isotope. α, β, γ indicate the type of radiation of natural and (α), (β), (γ) that of artificially produced radioactive elements.

Der Index links vom Symbol unten gibt die Ordnungszahl, der oben die Massenzahl des häufigsten Isotops an; α, β, γ ist die Art der ausgesandten Strahlung natürlicher, (α), (β), (γ) künstlich erzeugter Radionuklide.

L'index à gauche en bas du symbole est le numéro atomique, en haut le nombre de masse de l'isotope naturel le plus fréquent, α, β, γ indiquent le type de rayonnement d'un radioélément naturel et (α), (β), (γ) celui d'un radioélément artificiel.

El índice izquierdo inferior del símbolo es el número atómico, el superior el número másico del isótopo más fréquente. α, β y γ indican el tipo de radiación de los elementos naturales y (α), (β) y (γ) la de los elementos artificiales.

Lit.: 1. LANDOLT-BÖRNSTEIN: I. 5. Berlin: Springer 1952
     2. WANG, Y.: Handbook, Cleveland: Chemical Rubber Co. 1969

1.4 The chemical elements and their most important properties
Die chemischen Elemente und ihre wichtigsten Eigenschaften
Les éléments chimiques et leurs principales propriétés
Los elementos quimicos y sus propiedades más importantes

1. Symbol - Symbol - Symbole - Símbolo
2. Atomic number - Ordnungszahl - Numéro atomique - Número atómico
3. Atomic weight - Atomgewicht - Poids atomique - Peso atómico
4. Mass number and composition in % of isotopes - Massenzahl und %-Anteil der Isotope - Nombre de masses et pourcentage des isotopes - Número másico y porcentaje de los isótopos
5. Mean energy of K photons - Mittlere Energie der K Photonen - Energie moyenne des photons K - Energía media de fotones K:keV
6. Mean energy of L photons - Mittlere Energie der L Photonen - Energie moyenne des photons L - Energia media de fotones L:keV

1	2	3	4			5	6
H	1	1.008	1 99.985	2 0.015		(0.013)	-
He	2	4.003	3 10^{-4}	4 100		(0.025)	-
Li	3	6.939	6 7.42	7 92.58		0.054	-
Be	4	9.012	9 100			0.109	-
B	5	10.811	10 19.78	11 80.22		0.184	-
C	6	12.010	12 98.89	13 1.11		0.279	-
N	7	14.007	14 99.63	15 0.37		0.393	-
O	8	16.000	16 99.76	17 0.04	18 0.20	0.524	-
F	9	18.998	19 100			0.675	-
Ne	10	20.183	20 90.92	21 0.26	22 8.82	0.849	0.018
Na	11	22.990	23 100			1.04	0.031
Mg	12	24.312	24 78.70	25 10.13	26 11.17	1.25	0.048
Al	13	26.982	27 100			1.49	0.069
Si	14	28.086	28 92.21	29 4.70	30 3.09	1.74	0.136
P	15	30.974	31 100			2.02	0.169

Lit.: 1. LANDOLT-BÖRNSTEIN: Zahlenwerte und Funktionen, I, 5 Berlin: Springer 1952
2. STORM, E., ISRAEL, H.J.: L.A.-3753 UC-34 Physics 1967
3. WANG, Y.: Handbook of Radioactive Nuclides, Cleveland 1969

1	2	3	4				5	6
S	16	32.064	32 95.0	33 0.76	34 4.22	36 0.014	2.32	0.205
Cl	17	35.453	35 75.53	37 24.47			2.64	0.243
Ar	18	39.948	36 0.34	38 0.06	40 99.60		2.98	0.286
K	19	39.102	39 93.1	40 0.01	41 6.9		3.34	0.262
Ca	20	40.08	40 96.97 46 0.003	42 0.64 48 0.18	43 0.14	44 2.06	3.72	0.385
Sc	21	44.956	45 100				4.12	0.438
Ti	22	47.90	46 7.93 50 5.34	47 7.28	48 73.94	49 5.51	4.55	0.495
V	23	50.942	50 0.24	51 99.76			5.00	0.555
Cr	24	51.996	50 4.31	52 83.76	53 9.55	54 2.38	5.47	0.582
Mn	25	54.938	55 100				5.96	0.646
Fe	26	55.847	54 5.82	56 91.66	57 2.19	58 0.33	6.47	0.714
Co	27	58.933	59 100				7.00	0.785
Ni	28	58.71	58 67.84	60 26.23	61 1.19	62 3.66	7.56	0.859
Cu	29	63.546	63 63.09	65 30.91			8.14	0.937
Zn	30	65.37	64 48.89 70 0.62	66 27.81	67 4.11	68 18.57	8.74	1.02
Ga	31	69.72	69 60.4	71 39.6			9.37	1.11
Ge	32	72.59	70 20.52 76 7.76	72 27.43	73 7.76	74 36.54	10.01	1.21
As	33	74.92	75 100				10.69	1.30

1	2	3	4				5	6
Se	34	78.96	74 0.87	76 9.02	77 7.58	78 23.52	11.38	1.40
			80 49.82	82 9.19				
Br	35	79.90	79 50.54	81 49.46			12.09	1.50
Kr	36	83.80	78 0.35	80 2.27	82 11.56	83 11.55	12.84	1.61
			84 56.90	86 17.37				
Rb	37	85.47	85 72.15	87 27.85			13.60	1.72
Sr	38	87.62	84 0.56	86 9.86	87 7.02	88 82.55	14.39	1.84
Y	39	88.905	89 100				15.20	1.96
Zr	40	91.22	90 51.46	91 11.23	92 17.11	94 17.40	16.04	2.08
			96 2.80					
Nb	41	92.906	93 100				16.90	2.21
Mo	42	95.94	92 15.84	94 9.04	95 15.7	96 16.53	17.78	2.34
			97 9.46	98 23.78	100 9.63			
Tc	43	(99)					18.69	2.48
Ru	44	101.07	96 5.51	98 1.87	99 12.72	100 12.62	19.63	2.65
			101 17.07	102 31.61	104 18.60			
Rh	45	102.91	103 100				20.59	2.80
Pd	46	106.4	102 0.96	104 10.97	105 22.23	106 27.33	21.58	2.95
			108 26.71	110 11.81				
Ag	47	107.87	107 51.82	109 48.18			22.59	3.11
Cd	48	112.40	106 1.22	108 0.88	110 12.39	111 12.72	23.63	3.27
			112 24.07	113 12.26	114 28.86	116 7.58		
In	49	114.82	113 4.28	115 95.72			24.75	3.44

1	2	3	4				5	6
Sn	50	118.69	112 0.96	114 0.66	115 0.35	116 14.30	25.84	3.61
			117 7.61	118 24.03	119 8.58	120 32.85		
			122 4.72	124 5.94				
Sb	51	121.75	121 57.25	123 42.75			26.96	3.78
Te	52	127.60	120 0.09	122 2.46	123 0.87	124 4.61	28.12	3.96
			125 6.99	126 18.71	128 31.79	130 34.48		
I	53	126.90	127 100				29.29	4.14
Xe	54	131.30	124 0.10	126 0.09	128 1.92	129 26.4	30.49	4.33
			130 4.08	131 21.18	132 26.89	134 10.44		
			136 8.87					
Cs	55	132.91	133 100				31.72	4.52
Ba	56	137.34	130 0.10	132 0.10	134 2.42	135 6.59	32.99	4.72
			136 7.81	137 11.30	138 71.66			
La	57	138.91	138 0.09	139 99.91			34.27	4.93
Ce	58	140.12	136 0.19	138 0.25	140 88.48	142 11.07	35.59	5.14
Pr	59	140.91	141 100				36.94	5.35
Nd	60	144.24	142 27.11	143 12.17	144 23.85	145 8.30	38.31	5.56
			146 17.22	148 5.73	150 5.62			
Pm	61	(147)					39.72	5.79
Sm	62	150.35	144 3.09	147 14.97	148 11.24	149 13.83	41.16	6.02
			150 7.44	152 26.72	154 22.71			
Eu	63	151.96	151 47.82	153 52.18			42.63	6.25
Gd	64	157.25	152 0.20	154 2.15	155 14.73	156 20.47	44.13	6.49
			157 15.6	158 24.9	160 22.0			

1	2	3	4				5	6
Tb	65	158.92	159 100				45.66	6.73
Dy	66	162.50	156 0.05	158 0.09	160 2.29	161 18.88	47.23	6.99
			162 25.53	163 24.97	164 28.18			
Ho	67	164.93	165 100				48.82	7.23
Er	68	167.26	162 0.14	164 1.56	166 33.41	167 22.94	50.45	7.49
			168 27.07	170 14.88				
Tm	69	168.93	169 100				52.11	7.75
Yb	70	173.04	168 0.13	170 3.03	171 14.27	172 21.77	53.80	8.02
			173 16.08	174 31.92	176 12.80			
Lu	71	174.97	175 97.4	176 2.6			55.53	8.30
Hf	72	178.49	174 0.18	176 5.20	177 18.50	178 27.14	57.30	8.58
			179 13.75	180 35.24				
Ta	73	180.95	180 0.01	181 99.99			59.10	8.86
W	74	183.85	180 0.14	182 26.40	185 14.40	184 30.64	60.94	9.17
			186 28.41					
Re	75	186.2	185 37.07	187 62.93			62.81	9.47
Os	76	190.2	184 0.02	186 1.59	187 1.64	188 13.3	64.72	9.77
			189 16.1	190 26.4	192 41.0			
Ir	77	192.2	191 37.3	193 62.7			66.67	10.08
Pt	78	195.0	190 0.01	192 0.78	194 32.9	195 33.8	68.65	10.40
			196 25.3	198 7.2				
Au	79	196.97	197 100				70.68	10.72
Hg	80	200.59	196 0.15	198 10.12	199 17.04	200 23.25	72.75	11.04
			201 13.18	202 29.54	204 6.72			

1	2	3	4				5	6
Tl	81	204.37	203 29.5	205 70.5			74.85	11.37
Pb	82	207.19	204 1.54	206 22.62	207 22.62	208 53.22	77.00	11.72
Bi	83	208.98	209 100				79.19	12.07
Po	84	(210)	radioactive				81.43	12.42
At	85		radioactive				83.70	12.78
Rn	86	(222)	radioactive				86.02	13.15
Fr	87		radioactive				88.40	13.52
Ra	88	(226)	radioactive				90.81	13.90
Ac	89	(227)	radioactive				93.28	14.29
Th	90	232.04	232 100	radioactive			95.79	14.69
Pa	91	(231)	231 100	radioactive			98.35	15.10
U	92	238.03	234 0.01	235 0.72	238 99.27	radioactive	100.96	15.51
Np	93	(237)	radioactive				103.63	15.93
Pu	94	(242)	radioactive				106.35	16.08
Am	95	(241)	radioactive				109.14	16.80
Cm	96	(242)	radioactive				111.98	17.25
Bk	97	243	radioactive				114.89	17.71
Cf	98	244	radioactive				117.86	18.18
Es	99	−	radioactive				120.92	18.65
Fm	100	−	radioactive				124.05	19.14
Md	101	−	radioactive					
No	102	−	radioactive					
Lr	103	−	radioactive					
Ku	104	−	radioactive					
Ha	105	−	radioactive					
?	106	−	radioactive					

1.5 Most important elementary particles
Wichtigste Elementarteilchen
Principales particules élémentaires
Partículas elementales mas importantes

Group Art Groupe Grupo	Name Name Nom Nombre	Symbol Symbol Symbole Simbolo	Restmass Ruhemasse Masse au repos Masa en reposo m_o $kg \cdot 10^{-27}$	m_o/m_{eo} –	Charge Ladung Charge Carga	Energy Energie Énergie Energia $E=m_o c_o^2$ MeV	HL *) HWZ PDV PVM $s \cdot 10^{-9}$
Leptons Leptonen Leptons Leptones	Photon	γ	O	O	O	O	∞
	Neutrino	ν	O	O	O	O	∞
	Electron	e^-, β^-	0.00091	1	−1	0.511	∞
	Positron	e^+, β^+	0.00091	1	+1	0.511	∞
	Muon	μ^-	0.1884	206.78	−1	105.66	1525
Mesons Mesonen Mésons Mesones	Pion	π^o	0.2407	264.2	O	135.0	$6 \cdot 10^{-8}$
	π-Meson	π^+, π^-	0.2489	273.2	+1 −1	139.6	18
	K-Meson	K^+	0.8805	966.6	+1	493.8	0.06
	K^o-Meson	K^o	0.8874	974.2	O	497.9	$6 \cdot 10^{-2}$
Nucleons Nucleonen Nucléons Nucleones	Proton	p^+	1.6725	1836.1	+1	938.26	∞
	Neutron	n	1.6748	1838.6	O	939.55	700 s
	Deuteron	d	3.3443	–	+1	1875.5	∞
	Triton	t	5.0070	–	+1	2808.8	12.3 a
	α-particle	α	6.644	–	+2	3727.2	∞

*) HL = Half-live
   HWZ = Halbwertzeit
   PDV = Période demi vie
   PVM = Período de vida media

Lit.: 1. COHEN, E.R., DUMOND I.W.M.: Rev.Mod.Phys. 37, 537 (1965)
      2. EBERT, H.: Physikalisches Taschenbuch, Braunschweig:
         Vieweg 1967
      3. KOHLRAUSCH, F.: Praktische Physik, Bd. I - III, Stuttgart:
         Teubner 1968
      4. JAEGER, G., HÜBNER, H.: Dosimetrie und Strahlenschutz,
         Stuttgart: Thieme 1974

1.6 Range of electrons, protons, deuterons and α particles
Reichweite von Elektronen, Protonen, Deuteronen und α-Teilchen
Parcours des électrons, protons, deutérons et des particules α
Alcance de los electrones, protones, deuterones y particulas α

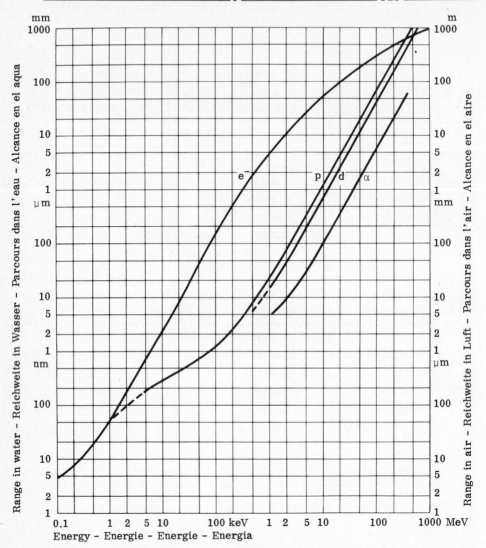

e⁻ : Electrons - Elektronen - Electrons - Electrones
p : Protons - Protonen - Protons - Protones
d : Deuterons - Deuteronen - Deutérons - Deuterones
α : α Particles - α-Teilchen - Particules α - Particulas α

Lit.: 1. LEA, D.E.: Actions of radiations on living cells, Cambridge:
          University Press 1946
       2. ROSSI, B.: High energy particles, N.Y., Prentice-Hall 1952
       3. HEISENBERG, W.: Kosmische Strahlen, Berlin: Springer 1953
       4. ICRU Report 16, Washington 1970

Energy Energie Energie Energía E	Range - Reichweite - Parcours - Alcance in - in - dans - en:				H_2O	Air Luft Air Aire
	e^-	p	d	α		
0.1 keV	4.5	–	–	–	mm	µm
0.2	8.0	–	–	–		
0.5	18	–	–	–		
1	53	(56)	–	–		
2•	170	(95)	–	–		
5	760	180	–	–		
10	2.5	280	–	–		
20	8.3	420	–	–		
50	42	750	–	–		
100	140	1.25	–	–		
200	500	2.4	–	–		
500	1.7	8.2	(6.0)	–		
1 MeV	4.3	22	16	4.5	µm	mm
2	10	80	45	9.4		
5	25	340	200	14		
10	55	1.2	750	105		
20	96	4.3	2.4	305		
50	190	19	12	1.7	mm	m
100	300	77	43	6.0		
200	480	250	150	22		
500	770	(1100)	730	(90)		
1000	1000	(3200)	(2300)	–		

The range of the particles in air is approximately 1000 times greater than that in water because the density of air is approximately 1/1000 that of water.

Die Reichweite der Teilchen in Luft ist wegen der gegenüber Wasser etwa 1000 mal geringeren Dichte rund 1000 mal größer als die in Wasser.

Le parcours des particules dans l'air est à peu près 1000 fois plus grand que dans l'eau puisque la densité de l'air est à peu près 1/1000 de celle de l'eau.

El alcance de las partícúlas en el aire es aproximadamente 1000 veces major que el correspondiente en agua, puesto que la densidad del aire es aproximadamente 1000 veces menor que la del agua.

1.7 Densities ρ of different materials
Dichte ρ verschiedener Stoffe
Densité ρ de différents matériaux
Densidad ρ de diferentes materiales

At - bei - à - a 20 - 25° C (1.013 bar = 760 mm Hg)

Elements - Elemente - Éléments - Elementos

Metals - Metalle - Métaux - Metales						Others - Andere - Autres - Otros		Gases-Gase Gaz-Gases	
Sym-bol	ρ (g/cm³)	Sym-bol	ρ (g/cm³)	Sym-bol	ρ (g/cm³)	Sym-bol	ρ (g/cm³)	Sym-bol	ρ (g/ℓ)
Li	0.53	Ni	8.90	Es	1.87	B	∿3.35	H	0.09
Be	1.85	Cu	8.96	Ba	3.5	C	1.8-2.3	He	0.18
Na	0.97	Zn	7.13	Ta	16.65	P	1.8-2.7	N	1.25
Mg	1.74	Ga	5.90	W	19.3	S	1.9-2.1	O	1.43
Al	2.70	Ge	5.32	Os	22.57	Br	3.12	Ne	0.90
Si	2.33	Se	∿4.5	Ir	22.42	Sb	6.22	Br	7.59
K	0.86	Sr	2.54	Pt	21.45	I/J	4.93	Ar	1.78
Ca	1.55	Y	4.47	Au	19.32			Kr	3.73
Ti	5.54	Mo	10.22	Hg	13.55			I/J	11.27
V	6.11	Pd	12.02	Tl	11.85			X	5.89
Cr	7.19	Ag	10.50	Pb	11.35	Air - Luft - Air - Aire			
Mn	∿7.3	Cd	8.65	Bi	9.75	760 mm Hg (= 1.013 bar)			
Fe	7.87	Sn_{gr}	5.75	Th	11.72	0° C			1.293
Co	8.9	Sn_{w}	7.31	U	18.95	20° C			1.205

Composite materials - Zusammengesetzte Stoffe - Materiaux divers - Sustancias compuestas	ρ g/cm³
Foam plastic-Schaumstoff-Plastique expansé-Espumas artific.	0.03-0.05
Cork - Kork - Liège - Corcho	0.22-0.26
Balsa wood - Balsa Holz - Balsa - Madera balsa	0.11-0.14
Soft wood - Weichholz - Bois tendres - Madera blanda	0.4 -0.8
Hard wood - Hartholz - Bois durs - Madera dura	0.7 -1.3
Plastics - Kunststoff - Plastique - Plásticos	0.9 -1.8
Sand,gravel - Sand,Kies - Sable,gravier - Arena,grava	1.6 -1.9
Brick massive-Ziegel massiv-Brique pleine-Ladrillo comp.	1.4 -2.2
Brick hollow-Ziegel hohl-Brique creuse-Ladrillo hueco	1.0 -1.4
Concrete, normal - Beton norm. - Béton norm. - Hormigón	1.5 -2.4
Concrete, heavy-Beton schwer-Béton lourd-Hormigón pesado	3.0 -6.0
Concrete foam-Schaumbeton-Béton expansé-Hormigón espumado	0.45-0.60
Paraffine - Paraffin - Paraffine - Parafina	0.87-0.91
Glass - Glas - Verre - Vidrio	2.4 -2.8
Flint glass-Bleiqals-Verre au plomb-Vidrio de plomo	3.3 -6.2
Soil (dry)-Erde (trocken)-Terre (sèche)-Tierra (seca)	1.3 -2.0

Liquids - Flüssigkeiten - Liquides - Líquidos	ρ g/cm³
Alcohol - Alkohol - Alcool - Alcohol	0.79-0.81
Ether - Äther - Ether - Eter	0.74
Glycerin - Glycerin - Glycérine - Glicerina	1.26
Gasoline - Benzin - Essence - Gasolina	0.66-0.69
Mineral oil - Erdöl - Huile minérale - Petróleo	0.81-0.85
Water - Wasser - Eau - Agua	1.00

Lit.: 1. WEAST, R.C.: Handbook of Chemistry and Physics, Cleveland, Ohio: CRC-Press 1974 - 1975
2. JAEGER, R., HÜBNER, W.: Dosimetrie und Strahlenschutz, Stuttgart: Thieme 1974

1.8 Linear energy transfer (LET) and specific ionization density
(ID) for different radiations in water (soft tissue)

Lineare Energieübertragung (LEÜ) und spezifische Ionisationsdichte (ID) verschiedener Strahlungen in Wasser (Weichgewebe)

Transfert d'énergie linéique (TEL) et densité d'ionisations
linéique (DI) pour differents rayonnements dans l'eau

Transferencia lineal de energía (TLE) y densidad de ionización específica (DI) en el agua, para differentes radiaciones

LET: energy transferred by a ionizing particle to matter along its
path in keV/µm. *)

LEÜ: von einem ionisierenden Teilchen in Materie entlang seiner Bahn
abgegebene Energie in keV/µm. *)

TEL: énergie transferée au milieu par la particule ionisante le long
de sa trajectoire exprimé en keV/µm. *)

TLE: energía transferida al medio por una partícula ionizada a lo
largo de su trayectoria, expresada en keV/µm. *)

ID: specific ionization density of ionizing particles in matter expressed in pairs/µm.

ID: spezifische Ionisationsdichte ionisierender Teilchen in Materie
ausgedrückt in Paaren/µm.

DI: densité linéique d'ionisation des particules ionisantes dans le
milieu, exprimée en paires d'ions/µm.

DI: Densidad de ionización específica de las partículas ionizadas
en el medio, expresada en pares ionicos/µm.

Terms used in graph and table - In der graphischen Darstellung und
in der Tabelle benützte Begriffe - Termes utilisées dans les
graphiques et les tables - Conceptos utilisados en el grafica y tabla

1. LET and ID of primary electrons of specific energy
   LEÜ und ID von Primärelektronen bestimmter Energie
   TEL et DI des électrons primaires d'énergie donnée
   TLE y DI de electrones primarios de energía determinada

2. LET and ID of electrons, including ionisation due to secondary
   electrons
   LEÜ und ID von Elektronen einschließlich der Ionisation durch
   Sekundärelektronen
   TEL et DI des électrons, y compris les ionisations dûes aux
   électrons secondaires
   TLE y DI des electrones incluyendo la ionización debida a elec-
   trones secundarios

3. LET and mean ID of electrons, integrated over the entire path
   length
   LEÜ und mittlere ID von Elektronen integriert über die gesamte
   Bahnlänge
   TEL et DI moyens des électrons intégrés sur la totalité de la
   trajectoire
   TLE y DI media de electrones, integrada sobre la longitud total
   de la trayectoria

*) For definitions see - Definitionen siehe - Pour les definitions voir - Para las
definiciones ver: ICRU Report No. 19, Washington D.C. 1971

4. LET and mean ID of electrons released by X-rays
   LEÜ und mittlere ID von durch Röntgenstrahlung ausgelösten Elektronen
   TEL et DI moyens des électrons mis en mouvement par les rayons X
   TLE y DI media de los electrones provocados por rayos X

5. LET and ID of protons of specific energy
   LET und ID von Protonen bestimmter Energie
   TEL et DI des protons d'énergie donnée
   TLE y DI de protones de una energía determinada

6. LET and ID of deuterons of specific energy
   LEÜ und ID von Deuteronen bestimmter Energie
   TEL et DI des deuterons d'énergie donnée
   TLE y DI de deuterones de una energía determinada

7. LET and ID of alpha-particles of specific energy
   LEÜ und ID von Alphateilchen bestimmter Energie
   TEL et DI des particules alpha d'énergie donnée
   TLE y DI de partículas alfa de una energía determinada

8. $\bar{E}$ mean energy of electrons released by monoenergetic X-rays
   $\bar{E}$ mittlere Energie der von monoenergetischer Röntgenstrahlung ausgelösten Elektronen
   $\bar{E}$ Energie moyenne des électrons mis en mouvement par les rayons X monoénergétiques
   $\bar{E}$ energía media de los electrones provocados por rayos X monoenergéticos

Energy of monoenergetic radiations - Energie der monoenergetischen Strahlungen - Energie des rayonnements monoénergétiques - Energía de las radiaciones monoenergeticas

Tube voltage for normal X-radiation - Röhrenspannung von Normalröntgenstrahlung - Tension normale du tube de rayons X - Voltaje del tubo par rayos X normales (see page - siehe Seite - voir page - ver página 70)

						keV/µm / n/µm			

LET, ID, and E at various particle energies E
LEÜ, ID und E bei verschiedener Teilchenenergie E   keV/µm
TEL, DI et E pour différentes énergies des particules   n/µm
TLE, DI y E para diferentes energías de las particulas

E *)	1 **)	2	3	4	5	6	7	8
LET – LEÜ – TEL – TLE: keV/µm								
keV								
1	6.2	8.4	13	13	–	–	–	1 keV
2	4.9	6.2	9.6	9.6	–	–	–	2 keV
5	1.95	3.9	5.9	5.9	–	–	–	5 keV
10	0.96	2.3	3.9	3.9	–	–	–	10 keV
20	0.55	1.3	2.2	2.6	–	–	–	15 keV
50	0.26	0.65	1.2	2.6	–	–	–	13 keV
100	0.16	0.39	0.72	2.3	–	–	–	16 keV
200	0.11	0.28	0.55	1.15	32	72	485	45 keV
500	0.065	0.18	0.39	0.49	17	36	260	140 keV
MeV								
1	0.060	0.19	0.31	0.32	9.8	21	160	350 keV
2	0.055	0.18	0.24	0.26	6.2	11.7	95	950 keV
5	0.060	0.18	0.21	0.23	3.1	6.2	49	3 MeV
10	0.065	0.19	0.21	0.23	1.95	3.7	29	7 MeV
20	0.068	0.20	0.22	0.22	1.14	2.3	18	15 MeV
50	0.080	0.21	0.23	0.23	0.58	1.10	9.2	36 MeV
100	0.094	0.24	0.26	0.26	0.32	0.65	4.9	70 MeV
ID – DI – DI – ID: n/µm *)**								
keV								
1	190	260	400	400	–	–	–	1 keV
2	150	190	290	290	–	–	–	2 keV
5	60	120	180	180	–	–	–	5 keV
10	30	70	120	120	–	–	–	10 keV
20	17	42	66	70	–	–	–	15 keV
50	8.0	20	35	70	–	–	–	13 keV
100	5.0	12	22	65	–	–	–	16 keV
200	3.2	8.5	17	38	1000	2200	15000	45 keV
500	2.0	5.6	12	15	530	1100	8000	140 keV
MeV								
1	1.8	5.7	9.5	10	300	650	4900	350 keV
2	1.8	5.7	7.5	8.0	190	360	2900	950 keV
5	1.8	5.7	6.5	7.0	95	190	1500	3 MeV
10	2.0	5.8	6.5	7.0	60	115	900	7 MeV
20	2.1	5.9	6.6	6.6	35	70	520	15 MeV
50	2.5	6.5	7.2	7.2	18	34	280	36 MeV
100	2.9	7.5	8.0	8.0	10	20	150	70 MeV

*)   E = Energy of the radiation – Strahlenenergie – Energie de la radiation – Energía de los rayos

**)   1 – 8 See pages – Siehe Seiten – Voir pages – Ver páginas 37–38

***)   n = Paires – Paare – Paires – Pares

Lit.: 1. GENTNER, W., MAIER-LEIBNITZ, H., BOTHE, W.: Atlas typischer Nebelkammerbilder, Berlin: Springer 1940
2. LEA, D.E.: Actions of Radiation on Living Cells, Cambridge 1946
3. CORMACK, C.V., JOHNS, H.E.: Brit.J.Radiol. 25, 369 (1952)
4. – 5.: WACHSMANN, F.: Strahlenther.86,440(1952); 89,128(1952)
6. ROSSI, B.: High energy particles, New York:Prentice-Hall (1952)
7. BURCH, P.R.J.: Brit.J.Radiol. 30, 524 (1957)

1.9 Physical units, constants and formulas
Physikalische Einheiten, Konstanten und Formeln
Unités, constantes et formules physiques
Unidades, constantes y fórmulas físicas

1. **SI basic units - SI-Grundeinheiten - Unités fondamentales SI - Unidades básicas SI**

Meter	Meter	Mètre	Metro	m
Kilogram	Kilogramm	Kilogramme	Kilogramo	kg
Second	Sekunde	Seconde	Segundo	s
Ampere	Ampere	Ampère	Ampere	A
Kelvin	Kelvin	Kelvin	Kelvin	K
Candela	Candela	Candela	Candela	cd
Mole	Mol	Mole	Mole	mol

2. **Units of force, pressure, energy, and power - Einheiten von Kraft, Druck, Energie und Leistung - Unités de force, de pression, d'énergie et de puissance - Unidades de fuerza, presión, energía y potencia**

Newton	1 N	=	$1 \text{ kg} \cdot \text{m/s}^2$
Dyne	1 dyn	=	$1 \text{ g} \cdot \text{cm/s}^2$
Torr	1 Torr	=	$1 \text{ mm Hg} = 1.333224 \cdot 10^2 \text{ N/m}^2$
Pascal	1 Pa	=	1 N/m^2
Joule	1 J	=	$1 \text{ W} \cdot \text{s} = 10^7 \text{ erg} = 6.2435 \cdot 10^{18} \text{eV}$
Calorie	1 cal	=	4.186047 J
Watt	1 W	=	$1 \text{ N} \cdot \text{m/s} = 10^7 \text{ erg/s}$
Bar	1 bar	=	$10^5 \text{ N/m}^2 = 10^6 \text{ dyn/cm}$

3. **Physical constants - Physikalische Konstanten - Constantes physiques - Constantes físicas**

Velocity of light
Lichtgeschwindigkeit
Vitesse de la lumière $\qquad c \quad = \quad 2.997925 \cdot 10^8 \text{ m/s}$
Velocidad de la luz

Electron charge
Elektrische Elementarladung
Charge de l'électron $\qquad e \quad = \quad 1.60210 \cdot 10^{-19} \text{ C}$
Carga electrónica

Planck's constant $\qquad h \quad = \quad 6.6256 \cdot 10^{-34} \text{ J} \cdot \text{s}$

Boltzmann's constant $\qquad k \quad = \quad 1.38054 \cdot 10^{-23} \text{ J/K}$

Avogadro's number $\qquad N_A \quad = \quad 6.02252 \cdot 10^{-23} / \text{mol}$

Loschmidt's constant $\qquad N_{L_2} \quad = \quad 2.6871 \cdot 10^{-19} / \text{cm}^3$

Mass-energy equivalent (= 1 kg)
Massenenergieäquivalent (= 1 kg)
Energie équivalente à une
masse de 1 kg $\qquad mc^2 \quad = \quad 8.98755 \cdot 10^{16} \text{ J}$
Energía equivalente de 1 kg
de masa

Dielectric constant
Dielektrische Konstante
Constante diélectrique $\qquad \varepsilon_o \quad = \quad 8.85419 \cdot 10^{-12} \text{ A} \cdot \text{s/V} \cdot \text{m}$
Constante dieléctrica

4. Decimal multiples and fractions - Dezimale Vielfache und Teile -
Multiples et sousmultiples décimaux - Múltiplos y submúltiplos
decimales

deca	da	10^1	deci	d	10^{-1}
hecto	h	10^2	centi	c	10^{-2}
kilo	k	10^3	milli	m	10^{-3}
mega	M	10^6	micro	μ	10^{-6}
giga	G	10^9	nano	n	10^{-9}
tera	T	10^{12}	pico	p	10^{-12}
peta	P	10^{15}	femto	f	10^{-15}
exa	E	10^{18}	atto	a	10^{-18}

5. Electric and magnetic units - Elektrische und magnetische Einheiten - Unités d'électricité et de magnétisme - Unidades eléctricas
y magnéticas

Ampere	1 A	=	1 C/s
Volt	1 V	=	1 W/A
Coulomb	1 C	=	1 A·S
Ohm	1 Ω	=	1 V/A
Farad	1 F	=	1 A·s/V
Henry	1 H	=	1 V·s/A
Weber	1 Wb	=	1 V·s
Oerstedt	1 Oe	=	$10^3/4\pi$·A/m
Gauss	1 G	=	10^{-4}Wb/m^2
Electrostatic unit	1 esu	=	$3.3356 \cdot 10^{-10}$ C

6. Mathematical formulas - Mathematische Formeln - Formules mathé-
matiques - Fórmulas matemáticas

Error analysis - Fehlerrechnung - Analyse d'erreurs - Análisis de
error

Arithmetic mean - Arithmetisches Mittel - Valeur moyenne -
Media aritmética

$$\bar{x} = \frac{1}{n} (x_1 + x_2 + \ldots + x_i + \ldots + x_n) = \frac{1}{n} \sum_{i=1}^{n} x_1$$

Mean-square error - Mittlerer quadratischer Fehler - Variance -
Error cuadratico-medio

$$s = \frac{1}{n-1} \sum_{i=1}^{n} (x_i - \bar{x})^2$$

Standard deviation - Standardabweichung - Ecart type - Desviación
standard

$$s_{\bar{x}} = \frac{s}{\sqrt{n}} \sqrt{\frac{1}{n(n-1)} \sum_{i=1}^{n} (x_i - \bar{x})^2}$$

41

7. Photon energies and wave lengths (λ) - Photonenenergien und Wellenlängen (λ) - Energie et longueurs d'onde (λ) des photons - Energías de los fotónes y longitudes de onda (λ)

Values rounded off - Zahlenwerte abgerundet - Valeurs arrondies - Valores redondeados

Photon energy - Photonenenergie Energie des photons Energía de los fotones			λ	Type of radiation Art der Strahlung Type de rayonnement Tipo de radiación
E	Joule	cal	nm	
1 eV	$1.6 \cdot 10^{-19}$	$3.82 \cdot 10^{-20}$	$1.24 \cdot 10^3$	Infrared-Infrarot
5 eV	$8.0 \cdot 10^{-19}$	$1.91 \cdot 10^{-19}$	$2.48 \cdot 10^2$	Visible light
10 eV	$1.6 \cdot 10^{-18}$	$3.82 \cdot 10^{-19}$	$1.24 \cdot 10^2$	Ultraviolet (UV)
50 eV	$8.0 \cdot 10^{-18}$	$1.91 \cdot 10^{-19}$	$2.48 \cdot 10^1$	
100 eV	$1.6 \cdot 10^{-17}$	$3.82 \cdot 10^{-18}$	$1.24 \cdot 10^1$	
500 eV	$8.0 \cdot 10^{-17}$	$1.91 \cdot 10^{-18}$	2.48	
1 keV	$1.6 \cdot 10^{-16}$	$3.82 \cdot 10^{-17}$	1.24	
5 keV	$8.0 \cdot 10^{-16}$	$1.91 \cdot 10^{-17}$	$2.48 \cdot 10^{-1}$	X- and γ-rays
10 keV	$1.6 \cdot 10^{-15}$	$3.82 \cdot 10^{-17}$	$1.24 \cdot 10^{-1}$	X- und γ-Strahlung Rayons X et γ
50 keV	$8.0 \cdot 10^{-15}$	$1.91 \cdot 10^{-17}$	$2.48 \cdot 10^{-2}$	Rayos X y γ
100 keV	$1.6 \cdot 10^{-14}$	$3.82 \cdot 10^{-17}$	$1.24 \cdot 10^{-2}$	"
500 keV	$8.0 \cdot 10^{-14}$	$1.91 \cdot 10^{-17}$	$2.48 \cdot 10^{-3}$	"
1 MeV	$1.6 \cdot 10^{-13}$	$3.82 \cdot 10^{-17}$	$1.24 \cdot 10^{-3}$	"
5 MeV	$8.0 \cdot 10^{-13}$	$1.91 \cdot 10^{-17}$	$2.48 \cdot 10^{-4}$	"
10 MeV	$1.6 \cdot 10^{-12}$	$3.82 \cdot 10^{-17}$	$1.24 \cdot 10^{-4}$	"
50 MeV	$8.0 \cdot 10^{-12}$	$1.91 \cdot 10^{-17}$	$2.48 \cdot 10^{-5}$	"
100 MeV	$1.6 \cdot 10^{-11}$	$3.82 \cdot 10^{-17}$	$1.24 \cdot 10^{-5}$	"

8. Temperature - Temperatur - Température - Temperatura

Kelvin   K $1 \text{ K} = -273.16 \text{ }^\circ C = -459.72 \text{ }^\circ F$

°Celsius   °C $x \text{ }^\circ C = (y \text{ }^\circ F - 32)/1.8 = x + 273.16 \text{ K}$

°Fahrenheit   °F $y \text{ }^\circ F = x \text{ }^\circ C \cdot 1.8 + 32 = x \cdot 1.8 + 241 \text{ K}$

Equivalent temperatures - Äquivalente Temperaturen - Températures équivalentes - Temperaturas equivalentes

°C	°F	°C	°F	°C	°F	°C	°F
-100	-148	-35	-31	± 0	+32	+40	+104
-90	-130	-30	-22	∓ 5	+41	+45	+113
-80	-112	-25	-13	+10	+50	+50	+122
-70	-94	-20	-4	+15	+59	+60	+140
-60	-76	-15	+5	+20	+68	+70	+158
-50	-58	-10	+14	+25	+77	+80	+176
-45	-49	-5	+23	+30	+86	+90	+194
-40	-40	±0	+32	+35	+95	+100	+212

Table of contents - Inhaltsverzeichnis
Table des matières - Tabla de materias

2.1 Radiological quantities and units
Radiologische Größen und Einheiten
Grandeurs et unités radiologiques
Cantidades y unidades radiológicas

2.1.1 Quantities - Größen - Grandeurs - Cantidades

Quantity Größe Grandeur Cantidad	Defining equation Definitionsgleichung Equation de definition Ecuación que las define	
Activity Aktivität Activité Actividad	$A = \dfrac{dN}{dt}$	Number of disintegrations dN/ time interval dt Anzahl von Zerfällen dN/Zeitintervall dt Nombre de désintégrations dN/ intervalle de temps dt Número de desintegraciones dN/ intervalo del tiempo dt
Absorbed dose Energiedosis Dose absorbée Dosis absorbida	$D = \dfrac{dW_D}{dm}$	Absorbed energy dW_D/mass dm Absorbierte Energie dW_D/Masse dm Energie absorbée dW_D/masse dm Energîa absorbida dW_D/masa dm
Absorbed dose rate Energiedosisleistung Débit de dose absorbée Indice de dosis absorbida	$\dot{D} = \dfrac{dD}{dt}$	Absorbed dose dD/time interval dt Energiedosis dD/Zeitintervall dt Dose absorbée dD/intervalle de temps dt Dosis absorbida dD/intervalo del tiempo dt
Exposure (Standard-)Ionendosis Exposition Exposición	$X = \dfrac{dQ}{dm_L}$	Induced charge dQ/mass dm_L of air Erzeugte Ladung dQ/Luftmasse dm_L Charge produite dQ/masse dm_L d'air Carga producide dQ/masa dm_L de aire
Exposure rate Ionendosisleistung Débit d'exposition Indice de exposición	$\dot{X} = \dfrac{dX}{dt}$	Exposure dX/time interval dt Ionendosis dX/Zeitintervall dt Exposition dX/intervalle de temps dt Exposición dX/intervalo del tiempo dt
Dose equivalent Äquivalentdosis Dose équivalente Dosis equivalente	$H = Q \cdot N \cdot D$ $D_q = q \cdot D$	Quality factor q x absorbed dose D Bewertungsfaktor q x Energiedosis D Facteur de qualité q x dose absorbée D Factor de calidad q x dosis absorbida D

Quality factors of different radiations
for radiation protection purposes:
Bewertungsfaktoren verschiedener Strahlen-
arten für Strahlenschutzzwecke:
Facteurs de qualité de différents rayonnements en vue de la radioprotection:
Factores de calidad de diferentes radiaciones para protección radiológica:

$$q$$
$$\beta, \gamma, \text{röntgen} = 1$$
$$n = 3 - 10$$
$$\alpha, p = 10$$

2.1.2 Units - Einheiten - Unités - Unidades

Quantity Größe Grandeur Cantidad	SI unit SI Einheit Unité SI SI unidad	Special name Besonderer Name Nom special Nombre especial (Symbol)	Non-SI unit Bisherige Einheit Unité hors système SI Unidad fuera de sistema SI
Activity Aktivität Activité Actividad	s^{-1}	becquerel (Bq)	curie (Ci) 1 Ci = $3.7 \cdot 10^{10} s^{-1}$
Absorbed dose Energiedosis Dose absorbée Dosis absorbida	$J \cdot kg^{-1}$	gray (Gy)	rad (rad) 1 rad = $0.01 \; J \cdot kg^{-1}$
Absorbed dose rate Energiedosisleistung Débit de dose absorbée Indice de dosis absorbida	$W \cdot kg^{-1} =$ $J \cdot kg^{-1} s^{-1}$	gray/s $(Gy \cdot s^{-1})$	rad/s (rad s^{-1}) 1 rad s^{-1} = $0.01 \; J \cdot kg^{-1} s^{-1}$
Exposure Ionendosis Exposition Exposición	$C \cdot kg^{-1}$	−	röntgen (R) 1 R = $2.5 \cdot 10^{-1} C \cdot kg^{-1}$
Exposure rate Ionendosisleistung Débit d'exposition Indice de exposición	$A \cdot kg^{-1} =$ $C \cdot kg^{-1} s^{-1}$	−	röntgen/s (R·s^{-1}) 1 R·s^{-1} = $2.5 \cdot 10^{-4} A \cdot kg^{-1}$
Dose equivalent Äquivalentdosis Dose equivalente Dosis equivalente	$J \cdot kg^{-1}$	−	rem (rem) 1 rem = $0.01 \; J \cdot kg^{-1}$

2.2 Radiological units formerly in use – Früher benützte radiologische Einheiten – Unités radiologiques anciennement utilisées – Unidades radiológicas empleadas anteriormente

Unit – Einheit / Unité – Unidad	Symbol / Symbole	Method – Methode / Methode – Método	Properties–Eigenschaften – Propriétés	Used–Gebraucht– Utilisées: in	Equivalent rad/unit
Sabouraud-Noiré	Sab	Change of color / Verfärbung / Variation de couleur	High energy dependence / Stark energieabhängig / Forte variation avec l'énergie	Europe 1915-25	~ 200 – 400
Holzknecht	H			Europe 1910-30	~ 50 – 200
Kienböck	X	Photographic	"	Germany 1920-30	~ 15 – 40
Fürstenau	F	Change of resistance	"	Germany 1920-30	~ 3 – 10
Solomon	R (French)	Ionization	Low	France 1925-35	0.4 – 1.2
Röntgen	R (German)	"	Wenig	World since 1930	$\approx$ 1.00
Röntgen	r (internat.)	"	Faible / Baja	World since 1930	0.88-0.96
Röntgen equivalent physical	rep	"	Also valid for $\alpha, \beta \ldots$ / Auch gültig für	USA since 1955	$\approx$ 1.00
Neutron	n	"	Valid for neutrons	USA since 1960	~ 1
Erythema dose	ED	Skin reaction / Hautreaktion	Inexact, but energy-independent	World since 1900	~ 600
Skin standard dose	HED (German)	Reaction cutanée / Reacción de la piel	Ungenau, aber energieunabhängig	Germany 1920-35	~ 800

Radioactivity – Radioaktivität – Radioactivité – Radioactividad

Unit	Symbol	Method	
Rutherford	rd	Disintegrations	$1\ rd = 10^6/s$
Stat	St	Ionization	1 St = amount of Rn 222 to produce $3.33 \cdot 10^{-10}$ A in air
mCi destroyed	mcd	"	1 mcd = 133 mgh with Rn 222
mg element h	mgeh/cm	"	1 mgeh/cm $\approx$ 6.5 rad
Eman	Eman	Disintegr./l	1 Eman = 0.275 ME (only Rn 222)
Mache	ME	"	1 ME = 3.64 Eman

Lit.: 1. ADLER, E.: Strahlenther. 5, 465 (1914) – 2. FÜRSTENAU, R.: Leitfaden, Stuttgart: Enke 1921
3. BEHNKEN, H., JAEGER, R.: Z.f.techn.Phys.7,563(1926) – 4. KÜSTNER, H.:Strahlenther.26,120(1927)
5. GREBE, L.: Strahlenther. 27, 358 (1928) – 6. HOLTHUSEN, H.:Grundlagen..., Leipzig:Thieme 1933
7. JAEGER, R., HÜBNER, W.: Dosimetrie u. Strahlenschutz, Stuttgart: Thieme 1974

2.3 Chemical composition and number of electrons/g of some materials and human tissues
Chemische Zusammensetzung und Elektronenzahl/g einiger Materialien und menschlicher Gewebe
Composition chimique et nombre d'électrons/g de quelques materiaux et des tissus humains
Composición química y número de electrones/g de algunas sustancias y tejidos humanos

Material / Materie / Matière / Material	ρ g/cm³	Proportion (weight) – Gewichtsanteile – Pourcentage (poids) – Porción en peso %									N_e $\frac{10^{23}}{g}$	1.	2.	3.
		H	C	N	O	Mg	P	Ar	Ca	Ti				
Air – Luft	$1.293 \cdot 10^{-3}$			76	23			1			3.01	0.499	3.67	223
H_2O	1	11			89						3.34	0.555	3.66	227
Graphite	2.25		100								3.01	0.500	3.00	108
Paraffin	0.88	15	85								3.45	0.573	2.70	92
Mix D	0.99	13	78		3	4				1	3.40	0.565	2.98	196
$(CH_2)n$	0.92	14	86								3.44	0.570	2.71	92.5
$(C_8H_8)n$	1.06	8	92								3.24	0.538	2.84	99.6
Perspex	1.18	8	60		32						3.25	0.539	3.16	147
Muscle–Muskel– Muscles–Musculos	1.05	10	12	4	73	0.4	0.2		0.01		3.31	0.549	3.60	230
Fat–Fett– Graisse–Grasa	0.92	12	77		11						3.36	0.558	2.87	111
Bone–Knochen– Os–Huesos	1.50	6	28	3	41	0.2	7		15		3.19	0.530	4.63	874

1. $(Z/A)_{eff}$ For Compton process and slowing down of electrons
Für Comptonprozeß und Elektronenbremsung
Pour l'effet Compton et le ralentissement des électrons
Para el proceso Compton y retención de electrones

2. $(Z^2/A)_{eff}$ For pair production and scattering of electrons
Für Paarbildung und Elektronenstreuung
Pour la production de paires et la diffusion des électrons
Para la formación de par y dispersión de electrones

3. $(Z^4/A)_{eff}$ For photoelectric effect – Für photoelektrischen Prozess
Pour l'effet photoélectrique – Para efecto fotoeléctrico

Z = Atomic number
Ordnungszahl
Nombre atomique
Número atómico

A = Atomic weight
Atomgewicht
Masse atomique
Peso atómico

N_e = Number of electrons/g
Zahl der Elektronen/g
Nombre d'électrons/g
Número de electrones/g

Lit.: 1. ATTIX, F.H., TOCHILIN, E.: Radiation Dosimetry, New York, London: Academic-Press 1969
2. JAEGER, R.G., HÜBNER, W.: Dosimetrie und Strahlenschutz, Stuttgart: Thieme 1974

2.4 Correction of the air density for ionization chambers
Korrektur der Luftdichte für Ionisationskammern
Corrections pour la densité de l'air pour chambres d'ionisation
Correcciones por densidad de aire en cámaras de ionización

The dose X_1, measured at air density ρ, (temperature t, pressure p) by means of an unsealed chamber which has been calibrated at ρ_0 (t_0, p_0) has to be corrected to yield the true value of X:

Die Dosis X_1, welche bei Luftdichte ρ (Temperatur t, Luftdruck p) mit einer nicht luftdichten Kammer gemessen wird, welche bei einer Luftdichte ρ_0 (t_0, p_0) calibriert wurde, muß korrigiert werden, um den wahren Wert X zu erhalten:

La dose X_1 mesurée avec une densité de l'air ρ (température t, pression p) au moyen d'une chambre non scellée étalonnée avec une densité de l'air ρ_0 (t_0, p_0) doit être corrigée pour obtenir la valeur vraie X:

Para obtener el verdadero valor de una dosis X, cuando la dosis X_1, ha sido medida por medio de una cámara no sellada a una densidad del aire ρ (temperatura t, presión p), calibrada a una densidad del aire ρ_0 (t_0, p_0), se debe corregir la lectura por medio de la siguiente fórmula:

$$X = X_1 \cdot \frac{\rho_0}{\rho} \qquad \rho = \frac{1.293}{1 + 0.00366\ t} \cdot \frac{p}{760} \ (mg/cm^3)$$

$$t\ (^\circ C) \qquad p\ (Torr)$$

Pressure Druck Pression Présion	Air density – Luftdichte – Densité de l'air – Densidad del aire								mg/cm³
	Temperature – Temperatur – Température – Temperatura °C								
Torr|mbar	0	5	10	15	20	25	30	35	40
640 853	1.089	1.069	1.050	1.032	1.015	0.997	0.981	0.965	0.950
650 866	1.106	1.086	1.067	1.048	1.030	1.013	0.996	0.980	0.965
660 880	1.123	1.103	1.083	1.064	1.046	1.029	1.012	0.995	0.979
670 893	1.140	1.119	1.100	1.081	1.062	1.044	1.027	1.010	0.994
680 906	1.157	1.136	1.116	1.097	1.078	1.060	1.042	1.025	1.009
690 920	1.174	1.153	1.132	1.113	1.094	1.075	1.058	1.041	1.024
700 933	1.191	1.170	1.149	1.129	1.110	1.091	1.073	1.056	1.039
710 946	1.208	1.186	1.165	1.145	1.125	1.107	1.088	1.071	1.054
720 960	1.225	1.203	1.182	1.161	1.141	1.122	1.104	1.086	1.068
730 973	1.242	1.220	1.198	1.177	1.157	1.138	1.119	1.101	1.083
740 986	1.259	1.236	1.214	1.193	1.173	1.153	1.134	1.116	1.098
750 1000	1.276	1.253	1.231	1.210	1.189	1.169	1.150	1.131	1.113
760 1013	1.293	1.270	1.247	1.226	1.205	1.185	1.165	1.146	1.128
770 1026	1.310	1.286	1.264	1.242	1.221	1.200	1.180	1.161	1.143
780 1040	1.327	1.303	1.280	1.258	1.236	1.216	1.196	1.176	1.157
790 1053	1.344	1.320	1.297	1.274	1.252	1.231	1.211	1.191	1.172
800 1066	1.361	1.337	1.313	1.290	1.268	1.247	1.226	1.206	1.187
810 1080	1.378	1.353	1.329	1.306	1.284	1.262	1.242	1.221	1.202
820 1093	1.395	1.370	1.346	1.322	1.300	1.278	1.257	1.237	1.217

1 Torr = 1.33 mbar
$^\circ C$ = K−273
$^\circ C$ = 5/9 · ($^\circ F$−32)

1 mbar = 0.75 Torr
K = $^\circ C$+273
$^\circ F$ = 9/5 · ($^\circ C$+32)

2.5 Energy- and photon fluence per röntgen
Energie- und Photonenfluenz pro Röntgen
Fluence en énergie et en nombre de photons par röntgen
Flujo de energía y de fotones por röntgen

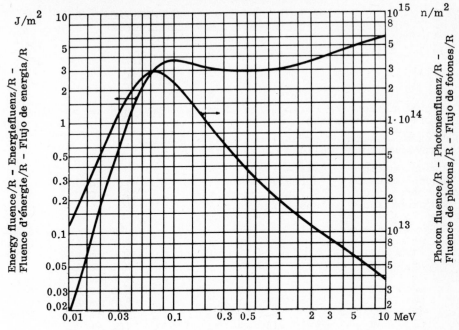

Energy - Energie - Energie - Energia

Photon energy Photonenenergie Energie des photons Energía de los fotones MeV	Fluence per röntgen - Fluenz pro Röntgen Fluence par röntgen - Flujo por röntgen	
	Energy Energie Énergie Energía J/m²	Number of photons Photonenzahl Nombre de photons Número de fotones n/m²
0.01	0.019	$1.18 \cdot 10^{13}$
0.02	0.170	5.31
0.04	1.301	20.30
0.06	2.849	29.70
0.08	3.576	27.90
0.10	3.714	23.20
0.20	3.243	10.10
0.40	2.946	4.60
0.66	2.956	2.79
0.80	3.007	2.35
1.00	3.126	1.95
1.25	3.267	1.63
2.0	3.714	1.16
4.0	4.672	0.73
8.0	5.717	0.447
10.0	5.993	0.375

49

2.6   Conversion of exposure to absorbed dose
          Umrechnung von Ionendosis in Energiedosis
          Conversion de l'exposition en dose absorbée
          Conversión de exposición en dosis energía

2.6.1   X- and gamma rays - Röntgen- und Gammastrahlung -
          Rayonnements X et gamma - Rayos X y gamma

2.6.1.1   Water - Wasser - Eau - Agua

Conversion factor - Umrechnungsfaktoren - Facteurs de conversion - Factores de conversión F_γ (rad/R)			
Radiation quality - Strahlenqualität - Qualité du rayonnement - Calidad de la radiación			
Monochromatic Monochromatisch Monochromatique Monocromática E_0	"Normal radiation" *) "Normalstrahlung" "Rayonnement normal" "Radiación normal"	HVL - HWSD CDA - CHR	F_γ rad/R
16 keV	32 kV	0.5 mm Al	0.89
21.5 keV	43 kV	1.0 mm Al	0.88
26.5 keV	53 kV	2.0 mm Al	0.87
35 keV	70 kV	4.0 mm Al	0.87
42.5 keV	85 kV	6.0 mm Al	0.88
50 keV	100 kV	8.0 mm Al	0.89
62.5 keV	125 kV	0.5 mm Cu	0.89
80 keV	160 kV	1.0 mm Cu	0.91
95 keV	190 kV	2.0 mm Cu	0.93
130 keV	260 kV	3.0 mm Cu	0.95
150 keV	300 kV	4.0 mm Cu	0.96
Cs 137	(Cs 137)	Cs 137	0.95
1 MeV	2 MV	–	0.95
Co 60	(Co 60)	Co 60	0.95
2 MeV	4 MV	–	0.94
3 MeV	6 MV	–	0.93
4 MeV	8 MV	–	0.93
5 MeV	10 MV	–	0.92
6 MeV	12 MV	–	0.91
7.5 MeV	15 MV	–	0.90
10 MeV	20 MV	–	0.90
12.5 MeV	25 MV	–	0.89
15 MeV	30 MV	–	0.88
17.5 MeV	35 MV	–	0.88

*) Definition "normal radiation" see page 70
   Definition "Normalstrahlung" siehe Seite 70
   Définition "rayonnement normal" voir page 70
   Definición "radiación normal" véase página 70

Lit.: 1. ICRU Report 23, Washington 1973

2.6.1.2 Ratio of mass absorption coefficients, tissue/air
Verhältnis der Massenabsorptionskoeffizienten Gewebe/Luft
Rapport des coefficients d'absorption massique tissu/air
Relación del coeficiente de absorción masico tejido/aire

$$\frac{(\eta/\rho)_{1-3}}{(\eta/\rho)_{air}}$$

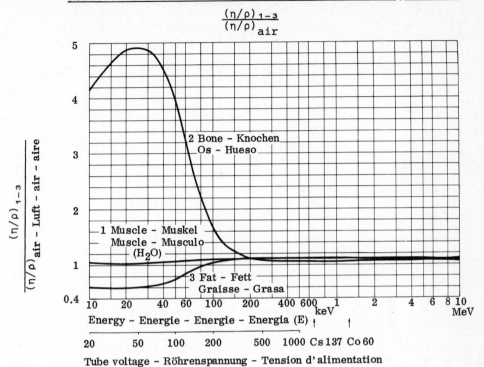

Energy - Energie - Energie - Energia (E)

Tube voltage - Röhrenspannung - Tension d'alimentation
Voltaje del tubo

E	$\frac{(\eta/\rho)_{1-3}}{(\eta/\rho)_{air}}$			E	$\frac{(\eta/\rho)_{1-3}}{(\eta/\rho)_{air}}$		
keV	1	2	3	MeV	1	2	3
10	1.04	4.17	0.61	0.2	1.11	1.12	1.11
15	1.01	4.59	0.59	0.3	1.11	1.08	1.12
20	1.00	4.81	0.58	0.5	1.11	1.07	1.12
30	1.01	4.86	0.59	Cs 137	1.11	1.06	1.12
40	1.01	4.55	0.64	1	1.11	1.06	1.12
50	1.03	3.97	0.74	Co 60	1.11	1.06	1.12
60	1.05	3.27	0.84	2	1.12	1.06	1.12
80	1.08	2.21	0.98	3	1.11	1.07	1.11
100	1.09	1.65	1.07	5	1.10	1.08	1.09
150	1.11	1.22	1.10	10	1.08	1.10	1.04

Lit.: 1. ATTIX, F.H., ROESCH, W.C.: Radiation Dosimetry, New York: Academic Press 1968
2. JAEGER, R., HÜBNER, W.: Dosimetrie und Strahlenschutz, Stuttgart: Thieme 1974

Corresponding values - Es entsprechen - Valeurs correspondantes
Valores corespondientes   in - in - en - en   1 Gy (= 100 rad)

Radiation HVL Strahlung HWSD Rayonnement CDA Radiación CHR	H$_2$O (Muscle Muskel-Muscle Musculo)		Bone Knochen Os - Hueso		Fat - Fett Graisse Grasa	
	R	C/kg	R	C/kg	R	C/kg
0.1 mm Al	111	$2.86 \cdot 10^{-2}$	28	$0.722 \cdot 10^{-2}$	187	$4.82 \cdot 10^{-2}$
0.5 mm Al	112	$2.89 \cdot 10^{-2}$	24	$0.619 \cdot 10^{-2}$	192	$4.95 \cdot 10^{-2}$
1 mm Al	114	$2.94 \cdot 10^{-2}$	24	$0.619 \cdot 10^{-2}$	196	$5.06 \cdot 10^{-2}$
2 mm Al	115	$2.97 \cdot 10^{-2}$	24	$0.619 \cdot 10^{-2}$	200	$5.16 \cdot 10^{-2}$
4 mm Al	115	$2.97 \cdot 10^{-2}$	24	$0.619 \cdot 10^{-2}$	187	$4.82 \cdot 10^{-2}$
6 mm Al	114	$2.94 \cdot 10^{-2}$	26	$0.671 \cdot 10^{-2}$	172	$4.44 \cdot 10^{-2}$
8 mm Al	112	$2.89 \cdot 10^{-2}$	29	$0.748 \cdot 10^{-2}$	156	$4.02 \cdot 10^{-2}$
0.5 mm Cu	112	$2.89 \cdot 10^{-2}$	38	$0.980 \cdot 10^{-2}$	137	$3.53 \cdot 10^{-2}$
1 mm Cu	110	$2.84 \cdot 10^{-2}$	53	$1.37 \cdot 10^{-2}$	120	$3.10 \cdot 10^{-2}$
2 mm Cu	106	$2.73 \cdot 10^{-2}$	65	$1.68 \cdot 10^{-2}$	110	$2.84 \cdot 10^{-2}$
3 mm Cu	105	$2.71 \cdot 10^{-2}$	83	$2.14 \cdot 10^{-2}$	106	$2.73 \cdot 10^{-2}$
4 mm Cu	104	$2.68 \cdot 10^{-2}$	94	$2.43 \cdot 10^{-2}$	106	$2.73 \cdot 10^{-2}$
Cs 137,1 MV,Co 60	105	$2.71 \cdot 10^{-2}$	110	$2.84 \cdot 10^{-2}$	104	$2.68 \cdot 10^{-2}$
2 MV	105	$2.71 \cdot 10^{-2}$	110	$2.84 \cdot 10^{-2}$	104	$2.68 \cdot 10^{-2}$
4 MV	106	$2.73 \cdot 10^{-2}$	111	$2.86 \cdot 10^{-2}$	106	$2.73 \cdot 10^{-2}$
6 MV	106	$2.73 \cdot 10^{-2}$	111	$2.86 \cdot 10^{-2}$	106	$2.73 \cdot 10^{-2}$
8 MV	108	$2.79 \cdot 10^{-2}$	111	$2.86 \cdot 10^{-2}$	108	$2.79 \cdot 10^{-2}$
10 MV	109	$2.81 \cdot 10^{-2}$	111	$2.86 \cdot 10^{-2}$	110	$2.84 \cdot 10^{-2}$
12 MV	109	$2.81 \cdot 10^{-2}$	110	$2.84 \cdot 10^{-2}$	111	$2.86 \cdot 10^{-2}$
15 MV	110	$2.84 \cdot 10^{-2}$	110	$2.84 \cdot 10^{-2}$	112	$2.89 \cdot 10^{-2}$
20 MV	111	$2.86 \cdot 10^{-2}$	109	$2.81 \cdot 10^{-2}$	116	$2.99 \cdot 10^{-2}$

Corresponding values - Es entsprechen - Valeurs correspondantes
Valores corespondientes   100 R (= $2.58 \cdot 10^{-2}$ C/kg)

Radiation HVL Strahlung HWSD Rayonnement CDA Radiación CHR	H O (Muscle Muskel-Muscle Musculo)		Bone Knochen Os - Hueso		Fat - Fett Graisse Grasa	
	rad	Gy	rad	Gy	rad	Gy
0.1 mm Al	90	0.90	361	3.61	53	0.53
0.5 mm Al	89	0.89	409	4.09	52	0.52
1 mm Al	88	0.88	424	4.24	51	0.51
2 mm Al	87	0.87	419	4.19	50	0.50
4 mm Al	87	0.87	409	4.09	53	0.53
6 mm Al	88	0.88	387	3.87	58	0.58
8 mm Al	89	0.89	343	3.43	64	0.64
0.5 mm Cu	89	0.89	266	2.66	73	0.73
1 mm Cu	91	0.91	187	1.87	83	0.83
2 mm Cu	94	0.94	155	1.55	91	0.91
3 mm Cu	95	0.95	120	1.20	94	0.94
4 mm Cu	96	0.96	106	1.06	94	0.94
Cs 137,1 MV,Co 60	95	0.95	91	0.91	96	0.96
2 MV	95	0.95	91	0.91	96	0.96
4 MV	94	0.94	90	0.90	94	0.94
6 MV	94	0.94	90	0.90	94	0.94
8 MV	93	0.93	90	0.90	93	0.93
10 MV	92	0.92	90	0.90	91	0.91
15 MV	91	0.91	91	0.91	89	0.89

2.6.2   Electrons - Elektronen - Electrons - Electrones

2.6.2.1   Water - Wasser - Eau - Agua

Depth / Tiefe / Profondeur / Profundidad	Conversion factor - Umrechnungsfaktoren - Facteurs de conversion - Factores de conversión C_e (rad/R)									
	Initial electron energy / Anfangsenergie der Elektronen / Energie initiale des électrons / Energía inicial de los electrones MeV									
cm	5	10	15	20	25	30	35	40	45	50
1	0.92	0.88	0.84	0.82	0.81	0.80	0.78	0.78	0.77	0.76
2	–	0.89	0.86	0.84	0.82	0.81	0.79	0.79	0.78	0.77
3	–	0.92	0.87	0.85	0.83	0.82	0.80	0.79	0.79	0.78
4	–	0.95	0.89	0.86	0.84	0.82	0.81	0.80	0.79	0.79
5	–	0.96	0.90	0.87	0.85	0.83	0.82	0.81	0.80	0.80
6	–	–	0.93	0.89	0.86	0.84	0.83	0.82	0.81	0.80
7	–	–	0.97	0.90	0.87	0.85	0.83	0.82	0.81	0.80
8	–	–	–	0.94	0.88	0.86	0.84	0.83	0.82	0.81
9	–	–	–	0.96	0.90	0.87	0.85	0.83	0.82	0.81
10	–	–	–	0.93	0.92	0.88	0.86	0.84	0.83	0.82
11	–	–	–	–	0.95	0.89	0.87	0.85	0.83	0.82
12	–	–	–	–	0.94	0.91	0.88	0.86	0.84	0.83
13	–	–	–	–	–	0.93	0.89	0.87	0.85	0.84
14	–	–	–	–	–	0.96	0.91	0.88	0.86	0.84
15	–	–	–	–	–	0.93	0.92	0.89	0.87	0.85
16	–	–	–	–	–	–	0.95	0.90	0.88	0.86
17	–	–	–	–	–	–	0.93	0.92	0.89	0.86
18	–	–	–	–	–	–	–	0.94	0.92	0.88
19	–	–	–	–	–	–	–	–	0.94	0.90
20	–	–	–	–	–	–	–	–	0.94	0.91
21	–	–	–	–	–	–	–	–	0.92	0.92
22	–	–	–	–	–	–	–	–	–	0.95
23	–	–	–	–	–	–	–	–	–	0.92
24	–	–	–	–	–	–	–	–	–	0.92

Lit.: 1. ICRU Report 21, Washington 1972

2.6.2.2 Stopping power ratios (S)
Verhältnis der Massenstoßbremsvermögen (S)
Rapport des pouvoirs d'arrêt massique (S)
Relación de la capacidades de frenado de masa (S)

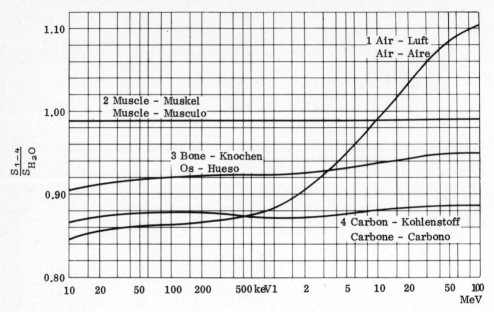

Energy - Energie - Energie - Energía

E	$\dfrac{S_{1-4}}{S_{H_2O}}$				E	$\dfrac{S_{1-4}}{S_{H_2O}}$			
keV	1	2	3	4	MeV	1	2	3	4
10	0.85	0.99	0.91	0.87	1	0.88	0.99	0.92	0.87
15	0.85	0.99	0.91	0.87	1.5	0.90	0.99	0.92	0.87
20	0.86	0.99	0.91	0.87	2	0.91	0.99	0.92	0.87
30	0.86	0.99	0.91	0.87	3	0.92	0.99	0.93	0.87
40	0.86	0.99	0.92	0.88	4	0.94	0.99	0.93	0.88
50	0.86	0.99	0.92	0.88	5	0.95	0.99	0.93	0.88
60	0.86	0.99	0.92	0.88	6	0.96	0.99	0.93	0.88
80	0.86	0.99	0.92	0.88	8	0.98	0.99	0.94	0.88
100	0.86	0.99	0.92	0.88	10	0.99	0.99	0.94	0.88
150	0.87	0.99	0.92	0.88	15	1.02	0.99	0.94	0.88
200	0.87	0.99	0.92	0.88	20	1.03	0.99	0.94	0.88
300	0.87	0.99	0.92	0.88	30	1.06	0.99	0.94	0.89
400	0.87	0.99	0.92	0.87	40	1.07	0.99	0.95	0.89
500	0.87	0.99	0.92	0.87	60	1.09	0.99	0.95	0.89
600	0.88	0.99	0.92	0.87	80	1.10	0.99	0.95	0.89
800	0.88	0.99	0.92	0.87	100	1.10	0.99	0.95	0.89

Lit.: 1. ICRP Report 21, Washington 1972

2.7   Change in radiation quality of X-rays with the depth
       Veränderung der Qualität von Röntgenstrahlen in der Tiefe
       Modification de la qualité du rayonnement X avec la profondeur
       Modificación de la calidad de rayos X con la profundidad

2.7.1 1 mm Cu HVL of the incident radiation - HWSD der einfallenden
       Strahlung - CDA du rayonnement incident - CHR de la radiación
       incidente

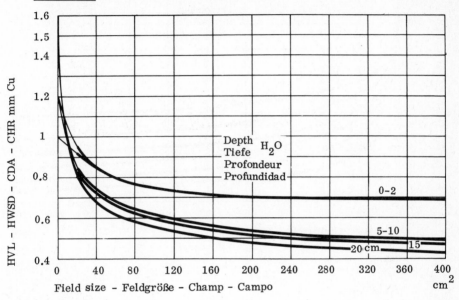

Field size - Feldgröße - Champ - Campo cm^2

2.7.2   2 mm Cu

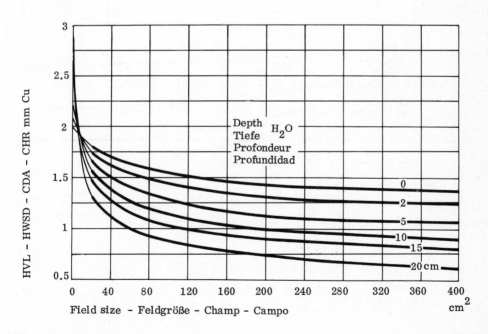

Field size - Feldgröße - Champ - Campo cm^2

2.7.3   4 mm Cu

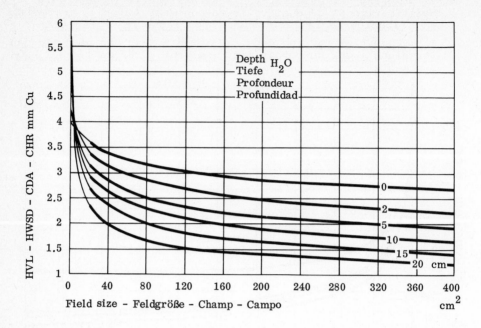

Field size - Feldgröße - Champ - Campo cm^2

2.7.4   Cs 137

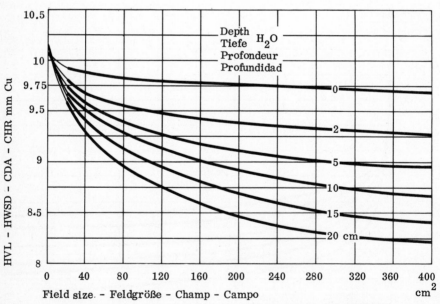

Field size - Feldgröße - Champ - Campo cm^2

Lit.: 1. LEGARE, J.M., GONCALVES da ROCHA, A.F.: J.Radiol.Electrol. 55, 495 (1974)

2.8 Evaluation of integral dose
Ermittlung der Integraldosis
Evaluation de la dose intégrale
Evaluación de la dosis integral

The integral dose, D_I, is the energy absorbed in the body of the patient and is expressed in g rad. For water-equivalent substances it can be calculated with sufficient accuracy for practical use according to the formula:

$$D_I = D \cdot F \cdot f_i \text{ (g R} \approx \text{g rad)},$$

where D = dose in R in the centre of the irradiated surface or, for radiations above 1 MeV, at the dose maximum;
F = irradiated area in cm^2 at the surface; and
f_i = integral dose factor, which can be obtained from the graph or from the table next pages.

In moving field therapy, D and F should be expressed in terms of equal SSD.

Die Integraldosis D_I ist die im Körper des Patienten absorbierte Energie und wird in g rad ausgedrückt. Sie kann für wasseräquivalente Körper mit praktisch ausreichender Genauigkeit nach folgender Formel berechnet werden:

$$D_I = D \cdot F \cdot f_i \text{ (g R} \approx \text{g rad)},$$

wobei D = die Dosis im Zentralstrahl an der Oberfläche bzw. bei Strahlungen über 1 MeV im Dosismaximum in R;
F = die bestrahlte Fläche in cm^2, an der Oberfläche und
f_i = der Integraldosisfaktor ist, der aus der Kurve oder Tabelle (siehe folgende Seiten) entnommen werden kann.

Bei Bewegungsbestrahlung D und F auf einen konstanten FHA beziehen.

La dose intégrale, D_I, est l'énergie absorbée dans le corps du malade et s'exprime en g rad. Pour les corps équivalents à l'eau, elle peut être calculée avec une précision suffisante en pratique, par la formule:

$$D_I = D \cdot F \cdot f_i \text{ (g R} \approx \text{g rad)}$$

avec D = dose en rad sur l'axe du faisceau à la surface, ou, pour les rayonnements d'énergie supérieure à 1 MeV, à la profondeur du maximum;
F = surface irradiée en cm^2 à la surface
f_i = facteur de dose intégrale relevé sur la courbe ci-jointe ou dans le tableau.

En radiothérapie cinétique D et F doivent être exprimé pour une même DSP.

La dosis integral D_I es la energía absorbida en el cuerpo del paciente y se expresa en g rad. Se puede calcular por cuerpos equivalentes al agua con suficiente exactitud práctica, medianta la siguien fórmula:

$$D_I = D \cdot F \cdot f_i \text{ (g R} \approx \text{g rad)}$$

donde D = dosis en el rayo central en superficie o, para radiaciones por encima de 1 MeV, en el máximo de dosis en R
F = area irradiada en cm^2 en superficie y
f_i = factor de dosis integral, que se puede sacar de la gráfica o tablas contiguas

En el caso de terapia de movimiento, D y F se referiran al DFP constante.

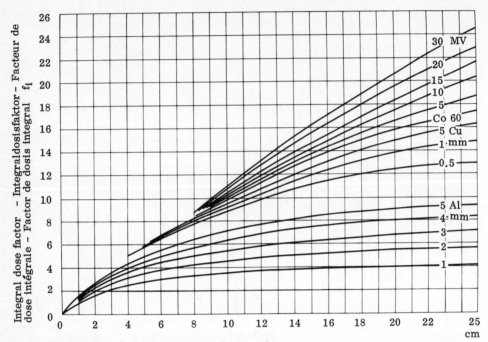

Integral dose factor – Integraldosisfaktor – Facteur de dose intégrale – Factor de dosis integral f_1

Thickness of the irradiated body (d)
Dicke des bestrahlten Körpers (d)
Epaisseur du corps irradié (d)
Espesor del cuerpo radiado (d)

Lit.: 1. MAYNEORD, W.V.: Brit.J.Radiol. 18, 12 (1945)
      2. WACHSMANN, F.: Strahlentherapie 93, 295 (1954)
      3. WATSON, T.A. et al.: Radiology 62, 165 (1954)
      4. KELLER, H.L.: Fortschr. Röntgenstr. 84, 73 und 85, 333 (1956)
      5. SCHOEN, D.: Strahlentherapie 120, 108/235/335/533 (1963)

d	Integral dose factors - Integraldosisfaktoren - Facteurs de dose intégrale - Factores de la dosis integral f_i							
	Radiation quality - Strahlenqualität - Qualité du rayonnement - Calidad de la radiación HVL - HWSD - CDA - CHR							
	mm Al					mm Cu		
cm	1	2	3	4	5	0.5	1	5
1	1.0	1.15	1.30	1.45	1.6	-	-	-
2	1.7	2.05	2.30	2.55	2.8	-	-	-
3	2.2	2.7	3.1	3.4	3.7	-	-	-
4	2.6	3.2	3.7	4.0	4.4	5.2	-	-
5	2.9	3.6	4.2	4.6	5.0	5.9	6.1	-
6	3.1	3.9	4.5	5.0	5.6	6.5	6.7	7.0
7	3.2	4.1	4.8	5.4	6.0	7.2	7.4	7.6
8	3.3	4.3	5.0	5.8	6.5	7.7	8.0	8.2
9	3.4	4.5	5.3	6.0	6.8	8.2	8.6	9.0
10	3.6	4.7	5.5	6.3	7.2	8.9	9.2	9.6
12	3.8	4.9	5.8	6.8	7.7	9.9	10.4	10.8
14	3.9	5.1	6.1	7.3	8.2	10.8	11.5	12.0
16	4.0	5.2	6.4	7.6	8.6	11.5	12.4	13.1
18	4.0	5.4	6.6	8.0	8.9	12.0	13.2	14.5
20	4.1	5.5	6.8	8.1	9.1	12.5	13.9	15.1
22	4.1	5.6	6.9	8.2	9.2	12.8	14.6	15.7
25	4.2	5.6	7.0	8.3	9.4	13.1	15.0	16.4

d	Integral dose factors - Integraldosisfaktoren - Facteurs de dose intégrale - Factores de la dosis integral f_i					
	Radiation quality - Strahlenqualität - Qualité du rayonnement - Calidad de la radiación					MV
cm	^{60}Co	5	10	15	20	30
8	8.5	8.5	8.6	8.6	8.7	8.8
9	9.2	9.3	9.4	9.6	9.8	10.0
10	9.9	10.1	10.3	10.5	10.9	11.1
11	10.6	10.9	11.2	11.5	11.9	12.1
12	11.3	11.6	11.9	12.3	12.9	13.4
13	12.0	12.4	12.8	13.2	13.9	14.4
14	12.8	13.2	13.6	14.0	14.7	15.4
15	13.4	13.7	14.3	14.7	15.6	16.4
16	14.0	14.5	15.0	15.6	16.5	17.3
17	14.5	15.0	15.5	16.3	17.3	18.2
18	15.0	15.6	16.4	17.3	18.1	19.0
19	15.5	16.3	17.1	17.8	18.9	19.9
20	15.9	16.7	17.5	18.5	19.6	20.8
21	16.2	17.1	18.1	19.0	20.2	21.5
22	16.5	17.5	18.7	19.5	21.0	22.2
23	16.9	18.0	19.3	20.5	21.7	23.0
24	17.2	18.4	19.9	21.2	22.4	24.0
25	17.4	18.8	20.4	21.9	23.0	25.0

2.9 Characteristics of various dosimeters – Eigenschaften verschiedener Dosimeter – Caractéristiques de différents dosimètres – Características de diferentes dosimetros

Suitable for – Geeignet für – Convenables pour – Apropiado para

System	Radiations / Strahlungen / Rayonnements / Radiaciónes (α β γ n)	Dose / Dosis / Dose / Dosis (1 2 3 4)	Dose rate / Dosisleistung / Débit de dose / Intensidad (1 2 3 4)	Accumulation / Speicherung / Intégration / Acumulación (5 6 7)	Error / Fehler / Erreur / Error (1 2 3)	Standard dosimetry	Energy dependence / Energieabhängigkeit / Variation avec l'énergie / Dependencia de la energia (1 2 3 4)	Detector size / Detektorgröße / Taille détecteur / Tamano detector (2 3)	Expenditure / Aufwand / Coût / Investición (2 3 4)
Ionisation									
Counter									
Calorimeter									
Chemical									
Photographic									
Radiophotolum.									
Thermolumines.									
Semiconductor									
Transparency									
Conductivity									
Scintillation									
Exoelectrons									

1. Very small/very good – Sehr klein/sehr gut – Três petit/três bon – Muy pequeno/muy bueno
2. Small/good – Klein/gut – Petit/bon – Pequeno/bueno
3. Medium – Mittel/mäßig – Moyen – Medio
4. Large–very large – Groß–sehr groß/schlecht – Grand–três grand/mauvais – Grande–muy grande/mal
5. Impossible – Nicht möglich – Imposible – Imposible
6. Limited possibility – Beschränkt möglich – Limitée – Limitado
7. Quite possible – Gut möglich – Possible – Muy adecuado

Lit.: 1. JAEGER, R.G., HÜBNER, W.: Dosimetrie und Strahlenschutz, Stuttgart: Thieme 1974

2.10 Practical hints for dose measurements

1. The functioning of the dosimeter (leakage and test reading) should be checked regularly. Temperature equilibrium between the chamber and the radioactive check source must be reached, and time for warmup must be allowed. Decrease in activity in the check source since reference date of the calibration protocol must be tanken into account. Tests for sensitivity, done with the check source should consist of several measurements; the relative standard deviation for 10 measurements should not exceed $\pm$ 0.5 %.

2. Measuring chambers should be chosen according to the purpose for which they will be used (energy range and dose range to be measured; directional dependence).

3. The method of measurement and the setup should be chosen correctly: Incident doses "in free air" should be measured without scatter from nearby objects. For low-energy radiations, absorption in air must be taken into account (see page 80); therefore it is recommended that measurements be made at the distance where the object is to be irradiated.

   The surface dose should be measured whith directionally independent chambers on the phantom surface (geometric center of the chamber at zero depth) or should be calculated from the incident dose by multiplication with the backscatter factor (see page 138).

   Reference doses are measured under specified geometric conditions in the phantom. A water phantom is recommended the sides of which are at least 5 cm from the beam edge and the height of which is at least 20 cm.

   Reference depths, according to recommendations by ICRU and DIN (1 - 4):

X- and Gamma Radiation		Electron Beams	
Peak energy	Depth	Incident energy	Depth
10 - 60 keV	0.5 mm	2 - 5 MeV	.5 mm
60 - 150 keV	5 mm	5 - 10 MeV	10 mm
150 keV - 3 MeV	50 mm	10 - 20 MeV	20 mm
>3 MeV	100 mm	20 - 50 MeV	30 mm

   Depth doses should be calculated from the measured surface doses or reference doses and from relative depth dose curves (see 86 and beyound. Note: Valid only for substances with water-equivalent absorption!).

   Tumor doses should be measured in the patient ("in vivo") at least occasionally, as a check for the correctness of the dose calculation, e.g., in the oral cavity, vagina, or rectum.

4. Measurements of radiation quality (HVL in mm Al or Cu) should be made in a narrowly collimated beam, with test filters located approximately halfway between the radiation source and the measuring chamber.

5. Correction of measurement results is neccessary if the conditions (energy, direction, field size, air density, etc.) differ from the calibration conditions.

Lit. see page 62

2.10 Praktische Hinweise für die Durchführung von Dosismessungen

1. Die Funktion des Dosimeters (Selbstablauf und Kontrollanzeige) regelmäßig überprüfen. Temperaturgleichgewicht Kammer/radioaktive Kontrollvorrichtung herstellen; Anwärmzeit beachten. Aktivitätsabnahme der Kontrollvorrichtung. Die Kontrolle der Empfindlichkeit mit der Kontrollvorrichtung sollte aus mehreren Einzelmessungen bestehen; die relative Standardabweichung sollte bei 10 Messungen nicht mehr als ± 0,5 % betragen. Prüfprotokoll berücksichtigen!

2. Meßkammern nach Verwendungszweck auswählen; Energie- und Meßbereich, Richtungsabhängigkeit usw. beachten.

3. Meßmethode und -anordnung richtig auswählen: Einfallsdosen "frei in Luft" ohne störende Streukörper messen. Bei weichen Strahlungen Luftabsorption berücksichtigen (siehe Seite 80), d.h. am besten im Bestrahlungsabstand messen.

   Oberflächendosis mit richtungsunabhängigen Meßkammern an der Phantomoberfläche (geometrische Mitte der Kammer in der Tiefe 0) messen oder aus der Einfallsdosis durch Multiplikation mit dem Rückstreufaktor (siehe Seite 132) berechnen.

   Bezugsdosen werden unter definierten geometrischen Bedingungen im Phantom gemessen. Hierzu wird ein Wasserphantom empfohlen, dessen Wände seitlich mindestens 5 cm vom Randstrahl entfernt sind und das eine Tiefe von mindestens 20 cm besitzt.
   Bezugstiefen nach Empfehlungen von ICRU und DIN (1 - 4):

Röntgen- und Gammastrahlung (Grenzenergie)		Elektronenstrahlung (Energie an der Oberfläche)	
10 - 60 keV	0,5 mm	2 - 5 MeV	5 mm
60 - 150 keV	5 mm	5 - 10 MeV	10 mm
150 keV - 3 MeV	50 mm	10 - 20 MeV	20 mm
>3 MeV	100 mm	20 - 50 MeV	30 mm

   Tiefendosen aus den gemessenen Oberflächen- oder Bezugsdosen und Kurven für die relative Tiefendosis (s. S. 86 ff.) berechnen (Achtung: Gilt nur für wasseräquivalent absorbierende Körper!).

   Herddosen wenigstens gelegentlich zur Kontrolle der Richtigkeit der Dosisberechnungen auch am Patienten ("in vivo"), z.B. in der Mundhöhle, im Ösophagus, der Vagina oder im Rectum, gemessen.

4. Messung der Strahlenqualität (HWSD in mm Al oder Cu) im eng ausgeblendeten Strahlenbündel mit Meßfiltern etwa in der Mitte zwischen Strahlenquelle und Meßkammer.

5. Korrektur der Meßergebnisse bei von Kalibrierbedingungen abweichenden Verhältnissen (Energie, Richtung, Feldgröße, Luftdichte usw.).

Lit.: 1.-4. ICRU Report 14 (1969), 17 (1970), 21 (1972), 23 (1973)
      5. MASSEY, J.B.: Manual of Dosimetry in Radiotherapy, IAEA Techn.Rep., Series 110, Vienna (1970)
      6. WACHSMANN, F., KALLERT, S.: Hdb.d.med. Radiologie, Band XVI/1, Heidelberg: Springer 1970
      7. PYCHLAU, P.: IAEA SM 84, 193 (1975)

2.10 Informations pratiques pour la mesure des doses

1 - Le fonctionnement du dosimètre doit être vérifié régulièrement
(fuite et tests de lecture). L'équilibre de température entre la
chambre et le dispositif radioactif de contrôle doit être établi
et un temps de chauffage suffisant doit être assuré. L'activité
du dispositif de contrôle doit être corrigée de la décroissance
et la validité du protocole de contrôle doit être vérifiée. Pour
tester la reproductibilité, plusieurs mesures devraient être
effectuées à l'aide du dispositif de contrôle; l'écart type ne
devrait pas être supérieur à $\pm$ 0,5 % pour 10 mesures successives.

2 - Les chambres devraient être choisies en fonction de la mesure
effectuée (domaine d'énergie, domaine de dose, réponse directio-
nelle, etc.).

3 - La méthode de mesure et le schéma de mise en place devraient
être choisis correctement: Les expositions "dans l'air" devraient être mesurées loin de tout diffuseur. Pour les rayonnements
de basse énergie, il est nécessaire de tenir compte de l'absorption dans l'air (voir page 80); il est donc recommandé que les
mesures soient effectuées à la distance à laquelle l'objet doit
être irradié.

La dose à la surface devrait être mesurée avec des chambres sans
effet directionnel, à la surface d'un fantôme (le centre géomé-
trique de la chambre étant à la profondeur O) ou bien elle devrait être calculée à partir de l'exposition dans l'air au moyen
du facteur de rétrodiffusion.

Les doses de référence sont mesurées dans des conditions géomé-
triques spécifiées, dans le fantôme. Il est recommandé d'utiliser un fantôme dont les bords soient à au moins 5 cm du bord du
faisceau et dont la hauteur soit d'au moins 20 cm.
Les profondeurs de référence suivant les recommandations de l'
ICRU (1 - 4) et de DIN sont:

Rayonnements X ou γ		Faisceaux d'électrons	
Energie maximale	Profondeur	Energie primaire	Profondeur
10 - 60 keV	0.5 mm	2 - 5 MeV	5 mm
60 - 150 keV	5 mm	5 - 10 MeV	10 mm
150 keV - 3 MeV	50 mm	10 - 20 MeV	20 mm
>3 MeV	100 mm	20 - 50 MeV	30 mm

Les doses en profondeur devraient être calculés à partir des
doses à la surface ou des doses de référence et des rendements
en profondeur (voir pages 86 ff). (Note: valables seulement pour
les substances équivalentes à l'eau.) Les doses à la tumeur devraient être mesurées dans le malade ("in vivo") au moins occa-
sionnellement, pour vérifier l'exactitude des calculs de dose,
par exemple, dans la cavité orale, le vagin, ou le rectum.

4 - Le mesures de qualité du rayonnement (CDA en mm Al ou Cu) devraient être faites dans des conditions de faisceau étroit, très
collimaté, et les atténuateurs devraient être placés à peu près
à mi-distance entre la source de rayonnement et la chambre d'
ionisation.

5 - La correction des résultats des mesures, lorsque c'est nécessaire, doit être faite si les conditions (énergie, direction,
champ, densité de l'air, etc.) différent des conditions d'
étalonnage.

Lit.: Voir page 62

2.10 Indicaciones prácticas para la realización de medidas dosimétricas

1. Comprobar periodicamente la función del dosímetro (control de aislamiento y medidor de control). Establecer el equilibrio térmico de la cámara/dispositivo de control radioactivo; préstese atención al tiempo de calentamiento. Tengase en cuenta la disminución de actividad del dispositivo de control y la validez del protocolo de prueba. Los controles de sensibilidad con el dispositivo de control deben de realizarse en varias medidas aisladas, la desviación standard relativa no debe ser superior a $\pm$ 0,5 % en 10 medidas.

2. Elegir las cámaras de medida de acuerdo con el fin práctico (intervalos de energía y medida, dependencia de la dirección).

3. Elección adecuada del dispositivo y método de medida: medir las dosis de inicidencia "libre en aire" sin cuerpos dispersantes perturbadores. Tengase en cuenta la absorción del aire en el caso de radiaciones blandas (vease pág. 80 o mejor aún medir a la distancia de radiación).

   Medir la dosis superficial con cámara de medida de dirección independiente en la superficie del muneco (centro geométrico de la cámara en profundidad 0) o calcularla multiplicando la dosis de incidencia por el factor de retrodispersión (véase pág. 132).

   La dosis de referencia se medirá en el muneco bajo condiciones geométricas definidas. Para ello se recomienda un muneco de agua, cuyas paredes se encuentren lateralmente del rayo marginal por lo meno 5 cm y que tenga una profundidad mínima de 20 cm. Profundidades de referencia según las recomendaciones de ICRU y DIN (1 - 4).

Rayos X y gamma (energía límite)		Radiación de electrones (energía en la superficie)	
10 - 60 keV	0,5 mm	2 - 5 MeV	5 mm
60 - 150 keV	5 mm	5 - 10 MeV	10 mm
150 keV - 3 MeV	50 mm	10 - 20 MeV	20 mm
>3 MeV	100 mm	20 - 50 MeV	30 mm

   Calcúlese la dosis en profundidad a partir de las dosis superficiales o de referencia medidas y las curvas de dosis en profundidad relativas (vease pág. 86 cont.). (Atención: Solo válido para cuerpo absorbente de equivalente acuoso!)

   Medir la dosis focal también en el paciente ("in vivo") p. ej. en la cavidad bucal, cuello de vagina o recto, al menos de vez en cuando, para controlar la exactitud de las medidas de dosis.

4. Medida de la calidad de la radiación (CHR en mm de Al o Cu) en haz de rayo estrecho atenuado con filtro de medida aproximadamente a la mitad entre la fuente de la radiación y cámara de medida.

5. Corrección de los resultados de medida correspondientes a las desviaciones de las condiciones de calibrado (energía, dirección, magnitud del campo, densidad del aire, etc.).

Lit.: Ver página 62

2.11 <u>What happens during irradiation of matter with 1 R (≈1 rad)?</u>
<u>Was geschieht bei Einstrahlung von 1 R (≈1 rad) in Materie?</u>
<u>Qu'arrive-t-il à un milieu irradié avec 1 R (≈1 rad)?</u>
<u>Que le sucede a la materia cuando se irradia con 1 R (≈1 rad)?</u>

$2.082 \cdot 10^9$ ion pairs/cm^3 in air (density 1.293 mg/cm^3)

$1.610 \cdot 10^{12}$ ion pairs/cm^3 in water

$3.34 \cdot 10^{-10}$ A per 1 R/s in 1 cm^3 air

$5.56 \cdot 10^{-12}$ A at 1 R/min in 1 cm^3 air

~ 84 erg/cm^3 water

$\sim 5 \cdot 10^{-6}$ (= 1/500,000) $^\circ$C heating of water

~ 1800 ion pairs/cell (assumed cell size: 10 x 10 x 10 μm= 1000 μm^3)

~ 225 ion pairs/cell nucleus (assumed size of cell nucleus: 125 μm^3)

~ 100 ionisations in a cell during passage of a non-densely
  ionising particle (X- or electron radiation), or

$\sim 10,000$ ionisations for densely ionising particles (α, p, or n);
  in the cell nucleus, ~ 50 or 5,000, ionisations respectively.

$\sim 3.5 \cdot 10^8$ ionisations per second, in a body of 70 kg, due to
  exposure to background radiation of 100 mR/year (~ 180 ionisations
  per cell per year).

$2,082 \cdot 10^9$ Ionenpaare/cm^3 in Luft (Dichte 1,293 mg/cm^3)

$1,610 \cdot 10^{12}$ Ionenpaare/cm^3 in Wasser

$3,34 \cdot 10^{-10}$ A je 1 R/s in 1 cm^3 Luft

$5,56 \cdot 10^{-12}$ A bei 1 R/min in 1 cm^3 Luft

~ 84 erg/cm^3 Wasser

$\sim 5 \cdot 10^{-6}$ (= 1/500.000) $^\circ$C Erwärmung von Wasser

~ 1800 Ionenpaare/Zelle (angenommene Zellgröße: 1000 μm^3)

~ 225 Ionenpaare/Zellkern (angenommene Größe der Zellkerns: 125 μm^3)

~ 100 Ionisationen in der Zelle beim Durchgang eines wenig dicht
  ionisierenden Teilchens (Röntgen- oder Elektronenstrahlung) bzw.

~ 10.000 dgl. bei dicht ionisierenden Teilchen (α, Protonen oder
  Neutronen); dgl. im Zellkern ~ 50 bzw. 5.000.

$\sim 3,5 \cdot 10^8$ Ionisationen/s in einem Körper von 70 kg Gewicht durch die
  natürliche Strahlenexposition von 100 mR/Jahr (~ 180
  Ionisationen/Zelle/Jahr).

$2,082 \cdot 10^9$ paires d'ions/cm³ d'air (densité 1,293 mg/cm³)

$1,610 \cdot 10^{12}$ paires d'ions/cm³ d'eau

$3,34 \cdot 10^{-10}$ A pour 1 R/s dans 1 cm³ d'air

$5,56 \cdot 10^{-12}$ A pour 1 R/min dans 1 cm³ d'air

~ 84 erg/cm³ dans l'eau

$\sim 5 \cdot 10^{-6}$ (= 1/500 000) °C élévation de température de l'eau

~ 1800 paires d'ions/cellule (taille moyenne de la cellule:
  10 x 10 x 10 μm = 1000 μm³)

~ 225 paires d'ions/noyau de cellule (taille moyenne du noyau de la
  cellule: 125 μm³)

~ 100 ionisations dans la cellule lors du passage d'un rayonnement
  faiblement ionisant (rayons X ou electrons)

$\sim 10~000$ ionisations pour des rayonnements fortement ionisants
  (particules α, protons ou neutrons); ~ 50 à 5 000 évènements dans
  les noyaux de cellule.

$\sim 3,5 \cdot 10^8$ ionisations/s dans un corps de masse 70 kg pour une exposition à l'irradiation d'origine naturelle de 100 mR/a. (~ 180
  ionisations/cellule/a).

$2,082 \cdot 10^9$ pares ionicos/cm³ en aire (densidad 1,293 mg/cm³)

$1,610 \cdot 10^{12}$ pares ionicos/cm³ en agua

$3,34 \cdot 10^{-10}$ A por cada 1 R/s en 1 cm³ de aire

$5,56 \cdot 10^{-12}$ A con 1 R/min en 1 cm³ de aire

~ 84 erg/cm³ en agua

$\sim 5 \cdot 10^{-6}$ (= 1/500 000) °C de calentamiento del agua

~ 1800 pares iónicos/célula (supuesto un tamaño de célula:
  10 x 10 x 10 μm = 1000 μm³)

~ 225 pares iónicos/núcleo celular (supuesto un tamaño de núcleo
  celular: 125 μm³)

~ 100 ionizaciones en la célula por el paso de una partícula poco
  ionizante (rayos X o radiación electrónica) o

~ 10.000 asimismo en el caso de partículas fuertemente ionizantes
  (α, protones o neutrones); asimosmo en el núcleo celular

~ 50 ó sea 5.000.

$\sim 3,5 \cdot 10^8$ ionizaciones/s en un cuerpo de 70 kg de peso mediante el
  efecto de la radiación natural de 100 mR/año (~ 180 ionizaciones/
  célula/año).

Table of contents - Inhaltsverzeichnis
Table des matières - Tabla de materias

3.1   <u>Relationship between tube voltage, filtration and HVL</u>
        <u>Zusammenhang zwischen Röhrenspannung, Filterung und HWSD</u>
        <u>Relations entre tension d'alimentation, filtration et CDA</u>
        <u>Relación entre la voltaje del tubo, filtración y CHR</u>

3.1.1   <u>10 - 150 kV Tube voltage - Röhrenspannung - Tension d'alimen-</u>
         <u>tation - Voltaje del tubo</u>

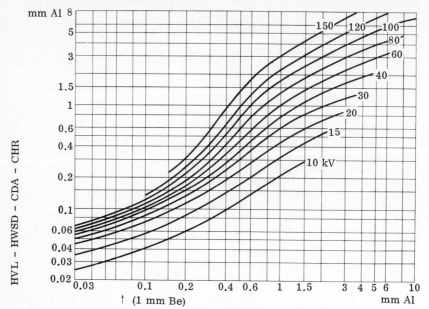

Filtration - Filterung - Filtration - Filtracion

Filtration Filterung Filtration Filtración total	HVL - HWSD - CDA - CHR mm Al							
	Tube voltage - Röhrenspannung - Tension d'alimentation - Voltaje del tubo kV							
mm Al	10	20	40	60	80	100	120	150
0.03	0.024	0.044	0.054	0.058	0.062	0.066	–	–
0.05	0.030	0.053	0.066	0.071	0.076	0.080	–	–
0.07	0.035	0.061	0.076	0.082	0.088	0.100	–	–
0.1	0.041	0.072	0.095	0.104	0.112	0.124	0.137	–
0.15	0.050	0.092	0.124	0.134	0.15	0.17	0.19	0.23
0.20	0.056	0.110	0.17	0.18	0.20	0.23	0.27	0.31
0.30	0.077	0.15	0.22	0.25	0.30	0.38	0.42	0.57
0.5	0.12	0.24	0.37	0.47	0.60	0.80	0.97	1.35
0.7	0.16	0.33	0.55	0.71	0.94	1.30	1.55	2.15
1.0	0.22	0.45	0.79	1.02	1.30	1.85	2.25	3.05
1.5	0.29	0.60	1.08	1.36	1.97	2.4	3.1	4.3
2.0	–	0.73	1.30	1.7	2.3	3.0	4.0	5.3
3.0	–	0.90	1.7	2.3	3.0	4.0	5.1	7.2
4.0	–	–	2.0	2.6	3.6	4.8	6.1	–
7.0	–	–	–	(3.4)	4.7	6.5	8.2	–
10.0	–	–	–	–	–	7.0	–	–

3.1.2 100 - 1000 kV Tube voltage - Röhrenspannung - Tension d'alimentation - Voltaje del tubo

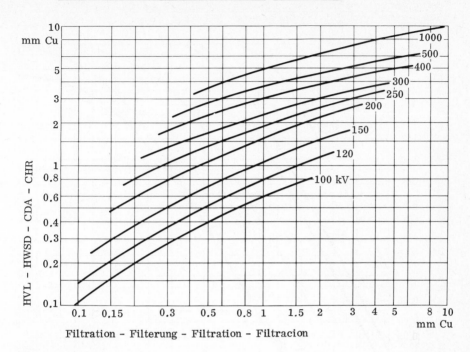

Filtration - Filterung - Filtration - Filtracion

Filtration Filterung Filtration Filtración total	HVL - HWSD - CDA - CHR								mm Cu
	Tube voltage - Röhrenspannung - Tension d'alimentation - Voltaje del tubo								kV
mm Cu	100	120	150	200	250	300	400	500	1000
0.1	0.105	0.145	–	–	–	–	–	–	–
0.15	0.155	0.21	0.295	0.48	–	–	–	–	–
0.2	0.20	0.26	0.38	0.59	0.81	(0.11)	–	–	–
0.3	0.28	0.37	0.51	0.80	1.10	1.40	1.80	(2.1)	
0.4	0.34	0.45	0.61	0.95	1.30	1.55	2.05	2.55	(3.2)
0.5	0.40	0.52	0.72	1.10	1.40	1.70	2.30	2.80	3.7
0.7	0.49	0.62	0.88	1.32	1.65	1.95	2.70	3.25	4.2
1.0	0.60	0.80	1.10	1.60	1.85	2.3	3.0	3.7	5.0
1.5	0.74	1.00	1.36	1.90	2.3	2.7	3.5	4.2	5.7
2.0	0.86	1.20	1.55	2.2	2.6	3.0	3.9	4.6	6.3
3.0	–	–	(1.8)	2.7	3.0	3.5	4.3	5.2	7.2
4.0	–	–	–	–	3.4	3.8	4.8	5.6	8.0
5.0	–	–	–	–	(3.6)	4.0	5.0	5.9	8.4
7.0	–	–	–	–	–	–	(5.3)	6.2	9.3
10.0	–	–	–	–	–	–	–	(6.7)	10.0

Lit.: 1. TROUT, D.E., GAGER, R.M.: Am.J.Radiol. 62, 91 (1949)
      2. - 3. ZIELER, E.: Strahlenther. 93,579 (1954); 100,595 (1956)
      4. HPA Report B, Series No. 7
      5. Authors' measurements - Eigene Messungen - Mesures personnelles - Medidas propias

3.2 "Normal radiation" and conversion from Al to Cu HVL
"Normalstrahlung" und Umrechnung von Al in Cu HWSD
"Rayonnement normal" et conversion CDA Al en Cu
"Radiación normal" y conversión CHR Al a Cu

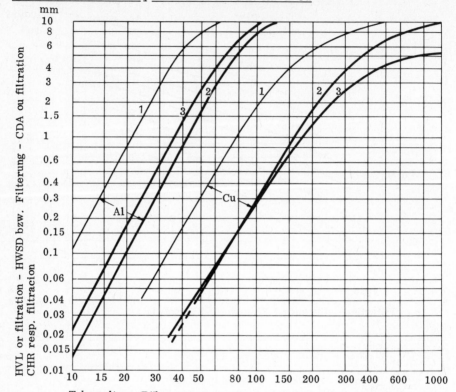

Tube voltage -Röhrenspannung-Tension d'alimentation-Voltaje del tubo
kV

1. Limiting value of the half-value layer (HVL) for monochromatic radiation
   Grenzwert der Halbwertschicht (HWSD), monochromatische Strahlung
   Valeur limite de la couche de demi-atténuation (CDA) pour un rayonnement monochromatique
   Valor límite de la capa hemirreductora (CHR) para una radiación monocromática

2. Half-value layer of the heterogeneous normal radiation
   Halbwertschicht der heterogenen Normalstrahlung
   Couche de demi-attenuation du rayonnement normal hétérogène
   Capa hemirreductora para la radiación normal heterogénea

3. Filtration required to produce "normal radiation"
   Erforderliche Filterung zur Erzeugung von "Normalstrahlung"
   Filtration nécessaire pour la production de "rayonnement normal"
   Filtración necesaria para la obtención de una "radiación normal"

Lit.: 1. WACHSMANN, F.: Strahlenther. 83, 41 (1950)
      2. DIN 6814, Bl. 2, Berlin: Beuth-Verlag 1970

"Normal radiation" - "Normalstrahlung" - "Rayonnement normal" - "Radiación normal" *)							
	HVL-HWSD-CDA-CHR mm Al		Filter Filter Filtre Filtro		HVL-HWSD-CDA-CHR mm Cu		Filter Filter Filtre Filtro
kV	1	2	3	kV	1	2	3
10	0.11	0.013	(0.022)	50	0.30	0.045	(0.05)
15	0.35	0.045	(0.075)	70	0.65	0.11	(0.12)
20	0.83	0.11	0.17	100	1.7	0.30	0.28
25	1.7	0.20	0.33	150	3.8	0.9	0.7
30	2.8	0.35	0.58	200	5.8	1.7	1.2
40	5.8	0.83	1.3	250	7.1	2.8	1.8
50	8.0	1.7	2.4	300	8.0	3.8	2.5
60	10	2.8	4.0	400	9.0	5.8	3.5
70	–	4.0	5.4	500	10	7.1	4.2
80	–	5.3	7.0	600	–	8.0	4.7
90	–	6.7	8.0	800	–	9.0	4.9
100	–	8.0	9.6	1000	–	10	5.1

*) "Normal radiation" means heterogeneous radiation which is filtered in such a way that its HVL is the same as that of homogeneous radiation of half the energy

Unter "Normalstrahlung" versteht man eine heterogene Strahlung, die so gefiltert ist, daß ihre HWSD gleich der einer homogenen Strahlung halber Energie ist

Par "rayonnement normal" on entend un rayonnement filtré de telle sorte que sa CDA soit égale à celle d'un rayonnement homogène ayant la moitié de l'énergie

Se denomina "radiación normal" a la radiación heterogénea que ha sido filtrada en tal forma que su CHR es idéntica a la de la radiación homogénea de la mitad de su energía

Conversion - Umrechnung - Conversion - Conversión: Al/Cu-Cu/Al **)							
HVL - HWSD - CDA - CHR:							mm
Al	Cu	Al	Cu	Cu	Al	Cu	Al
0.5	(0.016)	3	0.08	0.010	(0.30)	0.1	3.6
0.6	(0.018)	4	0.11	0.015	(0.48)	0.15	5.2
0.7	0.021	5	0.14	0.020	0.66	0.20	6.5
0.8	0.024	6	0.19	0.03	1.00	0.30	8.0
1.0	0.030	7	0.24	0.04	1.35	0.40	9.0
1.5	0.042	8	0.30	0.05	1.8	0.50	9.5
2.0	0.055	9	0.40	0.06	2.2	0.60	(10.5)
2.5	0.68	10	0.55	0.08	3.0	0.70	(11.0)

**) Valid only approximately and only for "normal radiations"
Gilt nur angenähert und nur für "Normalstrahlungen"
Valeur approchée valable seulement pour un "rayonnement normal"
Valor sólo aproximado y únicamente para "radiaciones normales"

3.3   X- and γ radiations for calibration
       Röntgen- und γ-Kalibrierstrahlungen
       Rayonnements X et γ pour l'étalonnage
       Radiaciones X y γ para la calibración

3.3.1 Radiotherapy dosimeters - Therapiedosimeter - Dosimétres
       pour radiothérapie - Dosímetros en radioterapia

3.3.1.1 Bremsstrahlung - Bremsstrahlung - Rayonnement de freinage -
        Radiación de frenaje

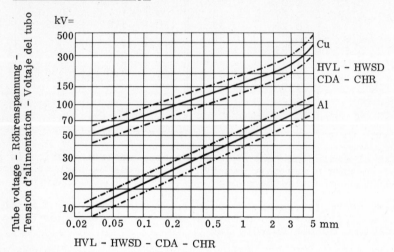

The radiations used for calibration should be similar to those used
in therapy. To accomplish this, one must choose those tube voltages
and filtrations which result in calibration radiations with HVL values that lie between the dashed curves.

Kalibrierstrahlungen sollen den in der Therapie verwendeten Strahlungen ähnlich sein. Um dies zu erreichen, müssen Röhrenspannungen und
Filterungen so gewählt werden, daß die erzielten HWSD der Kalibrierstrahlungen zwischen den strichpunktierten Kurven liegen.

Les rayonnements utilisés pour les étalonnages devraient être voisins
de ceux utilisés en thérapie. Dans,ce but, les tensions des tubes,
et les filtrations doivent être determinées de telle sorte que la CDA
se trouve dans la zône limitée par les courbes en pointillé sur la
figure.

Las radiaciones usadas para la calibración deben ser similares a las
usadas en terapia. Para obtenerlo, deben seleccionarse los voltajes
del tubo y ajustar la filtración hasta que la CHR se encuentre dentro
del área limitada por las líneas interrumpidas de la figura.

3.3.1.2 Radionuclides - Radionuklide - Radionuclides - Radionúclidos

                        ^{137}Cs; ^{60}Co

See also page - Siehe auch Seite - Voir aussi page - Ver también pagina 73

3.3.2　Radiation protection dosimeters
Strahlenschutzdosimeter
Dosimetres pour la protection
Dosímetros de protección

3.3.2.1　Narrow spectra (highly filtered radiation) - Hart gefilterte Strahlung - Spectres étroits - Espectros estrechos

Tube voltage Röhrenspannung Tension au tube Voltaje del tubo	Total filtration Gesamtfilter Filtration totale mm Filtracion total				Mean energy Mittlere Energie Energie moyenne Energia média	First HVL Erste HWSD Première CDA Primera CHR
kV=	Al	Pb	Sn	Cu	keV	mm
20	1	-	-	-	16	0.35 Al
30	4	-	-	-	25	1.20 Al
40	4	-	-	0.21	29	0.09 Cu
60	4	-	-	0.6	48	0.24 Cu
80	4	-	-	2.0	66	0.59 Cu
100	4	-	-	5.0	83	1.16 Cu
120	4	-	1.0	5.0	99	1.73 Cu
150	4	-	2.5	-	119	2.40 Cu
200	4	-	3.0	2.0	157	3.90 Cu
250	4	-	2.0	-	205	5.20 Cu
300	4	-	3.0	-	248	6.30 Cu

3.3.2.2　Wide spectra (radiation with low filtration) - Wenig gefilterte Strahlung - Spectres larges - Amplio espectro

Tube voltage Röhrenspannung Tension au tube Voltaje del tubo	Total filtration Gesamtfilter Filtration totale mm Filtracion total			Mean energy Mittlere Energie Energie moyenne Energia média	First HVL Erste HWSD Premiere CDA Primera CHR
kV=	Al	Sn	Cu	keV	mm
60	4	-	0.3	45	0.18 Cu
80	4	-	0.5	58	0.35 Cu
110	4	-	2.0	79	0.94 Cu
150	4	1.0	-	104	1.86 Cu
200	4	2.0	-	134	3.11 Cu
250	4	4.0	-	169	4.3 Cu
300	4	6.5	-	202	5.0 Cu

3.3.2.3　Radionuclides - Radionuklide - Radionuclides - Radionuclidos

Nuclide Nuklid Nucléide Nucléido	Energy Energie γ Energie Energía	Half-life Halbwertzeit Période Periodo	Gamma-ray constant Gammastrahlenkonstante Γ Constante spécifique Constante específica	
			$R\ m^2h^{-1}Ci^{-1}$	$C\ m^2kg^{-1}$
$^{125}I\ ^{125}J$	35 keV	60.1 d	0.0044	$0.084 \cdot 10^{18}$
^{241}Am	60 keV	458 a	0.013	0.025 "
^{57}Co	122 keV	270.5 d	0.097	0.186 "
^{203}Hg	279 keV	47 d	0.119	0.285 "
^{137}Cs	662 keV	29.9 a	0.336	0.626 "
^{60}Co	1.25 MeV	5.272 a	1.31	2.52 "

Lit.: 1. DREXLER, G., GOSSRAU, M.: IAEA-SM 143, 16 (1971)
2. ISO TC 62, Draft May 1974
3. DIN 6818, Berlin: Beuth-Verlag, Entwurf Nov. 1974

3.4　Exposure rate for different voltages and filtrations
Dosisleistungen bei verschiedenen Spannungen und Filterungen
Débit d'exposition pour différentes tensions et filtrations
Indice de exposición con diferentes voltajes y filtros

3.4.1　10 - 150 kV Voltage range - Spannungsbereich - Domaine de
tensions - Gama de kilovoltaje

0.02 - 8 mm Al Filtration-Filterung-Filtration-Filtración

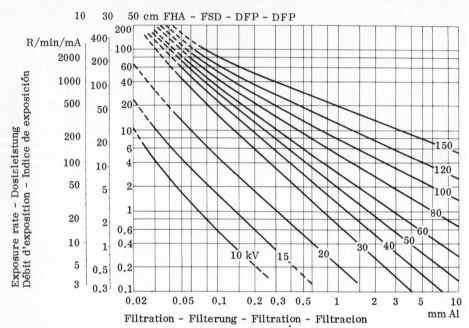

The average values given are for DC voltage and for an anode
angle of 45° (therapy tubes). For voltages with greater fluctuation
(see also page 79), and for smaller anode angles (diagnostic tubes),
the exposure rates are 20 - 40 % lower (also valid for page 76).

Die angegebenen Richtwerte gelten für Gleichspannung und Anodenwin-
kel von 45° (Therapieröhren). Bei Spannungen größerer Welligkeit
(siehe auch Seite 79) und kleineren Anodenwinkeln (Diagnostikröhren)
liegen die Dosisleistungen um 20 - 40 % niedriger (gilt auch für
Seite 76).

Valeurs moyennes données pour des tensions constantes et pour une
anode à 45° (tubes de thérapie). Pour des tensions pulsatoires et
pour des anodes avec des angles plus faibles (tubes de diagnostic)
les débits d'exposition sont 20 à 40 % plus faibles (vaut également
pour page 76).

Los valores estimativos indicados son válidos para corriente continua y ángulo de ánodo de 45° (tubos de terapía). Para voltajes de
mayor fluctuación (véase también página 79) y ángulos anódicos
menores (tubos de diagnóstico) las intensidades de dosis son un
20 - 40 % inferiores (vale también para página 76).

Lit.: 1. JENNINGS, W.A.: Cathode Press 7, 28 (1949/50)
      2. WACHSMANN, F.: Strahlenther. 83, 41 (1950)
      3. Mc CULLOUGH, E.C., CAMERON, R.: Brit.J.Radiol. 43,448 (1970)

FSD FHA DFP DFP	Filter Filter Filtre Filtro mm Al	Exposure rate - Dosisleistung / Débit d'exposition - Indice de exposición — R/min mA							
		Tube voltage - Röhrenspannung / Tension d'alimentation - Voltaje del tubo — kV=							
	Al	10	20	40	60	80	100	120	150
10 cm	0.02	(275)	(1600)	-	-	-	-	-	-
	0.03	(300)	(750)	(3300)	-	-	-	-	-
	0.04	(60)	(470)	(2100)	(2800)	-	-	-	-
	0.06	(30)	250	1100	(1600)	(2000)	-	-	-
	0.08	20	160	770	1100	1400	-	-	-
	0.1	12	110	580	880	1050	(1300)	-	-
	0.2	(5.0)	45	225	400	550	700	-	-
	0.3	-	25	140	250	375	500	(720)	-
	0.4	-	18	100	190	275	375	570	-
	0.6	-	10	58	125	200	275	450	(670)
	0.8	-	7.0	40	90	150	225	360	560
	1	-	5.0	30	72	125	200	300	500
	2	-	-	12	35	68	110	190	350
	3	-	-	7.5	23	48	85	140	250
	4	-	-	5.2	18	35	70	110	220
	6	-	-	3.2	12	25	50	85	170
	8	-	-	-	8.2	20	40	68	145
30 cm	0.02	(15)	(130)	-	-	-	-	-	-
	0.03	(17)	(70)	(310)	-	-	-	-	-
	0.04	(4.0)	(45)	(200)	(260)	(320)	(380)	-	-
	0.06	2.0	22	110	160	(200)	225	(320)	-
	0.08	1.5	13	75	110	130	160	(240)	
	0.1	0.9	11	60	95	105	140	(200)	(275)
	0.2	(0.5)	4.7	24	45	60	75	(110)	(180)
	0.3	-	2.9	15	28	42	54	80	110
	0.4	-	2.0	11	21	30	42	62	92
	0.6	-	1.1	6.2	14	22	30	48	75
	0.8	-	0.8	4.4	10	16	25	40	62
	1	-	0.5	3.3	8.0	14	22	34	55
	2	-	-	1.3	3.8	7.5	12	21	40
	3	-	-	0.8	2.5	4.2	9.5	16	28
	4	-	-	0.5	2.0	3.8	7.8	12	24
	6	-	-	0.3	1.3	2.7	5.5	10	19
	8	-	-	-	0.9	2.2	4.4	8.0	16
50 cm	0.02	(3.5)	(32)	-	-	-	-	-	-
	0.04	(1.0)	(16)	(60)	(90)	(110)	(150)	-	-
	0.06	0.5	(11)	(36)	(52)	(66)	90	105	150
	0.08	0.4	5.5	25	36	47	64	80	105
	0.1	0.25	3.8	15	28	35	45	64	90
	0.2	(0.15)	1.2	7.5	14	20	25	38	62
	0.3	-	0.9	5.0	9.4	14	19	28	40
	0.4	-	0.6	3.8	7.0	11	14	22	33
	0.6	-	0.4	2.2	4.7	7.8	10	17	26
	0.8	-	0.3	1.5	3.5	5.8	8.6	14	22
	1	-	0.2	1.3	2.8	4.8	7.8	12	20
	2	-	-	0.4	1.3	2.7	4.2	7.2	14
	3	-	-	0.3	0.9	2.0	3.4	5.7	10
	4	-	-	0.2	0.7	1.4	2.8	4.3	8.5
	6	-	-	0.1	0.5	1.0	2.0	3.5	6.8
	8	-	-	-	0.3	0.8	1.6	2.8	5.8

3.4.2 <u>60 - 500 kV Voltage range - Spannungsbereich -</u>
<u>Domaine de tensions - Gama de kilovoltaje</u>

Cu Filtration - Filterung - Filtration - Filtración

30 - 50 - 80 cm FSD - FHA - DFP - DFP

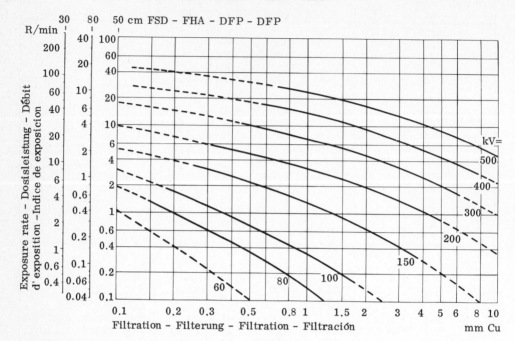

In half wave and fully rectified operation, the exposure rates on the
same peak voltages are approximately half of the values given above.

Im Ein- oder Zweipulsbetrieb der Röntgenröhre sind die Dosisleistungen bezogen auf gleiche Scheitelspannungen etwa halb so groß wie angegeben.

Pour le fonctionnement en une ou deux alternances les débits d'exposition sont environ la moitié de ceux indiqués pour la même tension de crête.

En el caso de que el aparato trabaje con semi-onda, los indices de
exposición se reducen, aceptando los mismos voltajes pico, aproximadamente a la mitad de aquellos dados.

Lit.: 1. DRESSER, R., COSMAN, B.J.: Am.J.Roentgenol. <u>39</u>, 972 (1938)
      2. TRUMP, J.G., van de GRAAF: Phys.Rev. <u>55</u>, 676 (1939)
      3. TAYLOR, L.S.: Medical Physics 2, 901 (1950)
      4. FARR, R.F.: Acta Radiol. <u>43</u>, 152 (1955)
      5. ICRP Publication <u>3</u>, Pergamon Press (1960)
      6. OSBORNE, S.B.: X-ray Focus <u>3</u>, 22 (1962)
      7. NCRP Publications, Report No. 33, Washington D.C. (1968)
      8. Mc CULLOUGH, E.C., CAMERON, J.R.: Br.J.Radiol. <u>43</u>,448 (1970)
      9. The Hospital Physicists' Association, Report No. 7 (1972)
     10. ICRP Publication <u>21</u>, External Sources, Pergamon Press (1973)
     11. DIN 6812, Berlin: Beuth-Verlag, Entwurf Februar 1974

FSD FHA DFP DFP	Filter Filtre Filtro mm Cu	Exposure rate - Dosisleistung Débit d'exposition - Indice de exposition Tube voltage - Röhrenspannung Tension d'alimentation - Voltaje del tubo 80	100	150	200	300	400	R/min 1 mA kV 500
	0.1	(5.3)	(8.2)	(14.5)	(25)	(48)	–	–
	0.2	2.6	4.8	(12.3)	(20)	(39)	(66)	(105)
	0.3	1.8	3.3	8.6	16	(34)	(56)	(98)
	0.4	1.2	2.6	7.2	14	(32)	(52)	(88)
	0.5	0.97	2.0	6.0	13	28	50	(80)
	0.6	0.77	1.6	5.2	11.5	25	47	75
	0.8	0.52	1.2	4.4	10.2	22	42	68
30 cm	1	0.38	0.96	3.7	8.8	19	39	62
	1.5	–	0.55	2.4	6.6	15	32	53
	2	–	(0.39)	1.8	5.2	13	25	43
	2.5	–	0.28	1.4	4.4	10.7	21	40
	3	–	–	1.15	3.8	9.1	18	36
	4	–	–	0.80	3.0	7.2	15	30
	5	–	–	0.57	2.3	5.5	12	24
	6	–	–	0.44	(1.8)	4.7	10.5	21
	8	–	–	0.28	(1.3)	(3.6)	7.7	16
	10	–	–	–	(0.94)	(2.8)	(6.4)	13
	0.1	(1.9)	(3.0)	(5.2)	(9.2)	(17.5)	–	–
	0.2	0.95	1.75	(4.5)	(7.2)	(14.0)	(24)	(44)
	0.3	0.63	1.20	3.1	5.9	(12.5)	(20)	(36)
	0.4	0.45	0.92	2.6	5.1	(11.5)	(19)	(33)
	0.5	0.35	0.72	2.2	4.8	10.0	18	31
	0.6	0.28	0.58	1.9	4.2	9.0	17	29
	0.8	0.19	0.43	1.6	3.7	7.8	15	26
50 cm	1	0.14	0.35	1.35	3.2	7.0	14	24
	1.5	–	0.20	0.88	2.4	5.4	11.5	19
	2	–	(0.14)	0.65	1.9	4.6	8.8	16
	2.5	–	(0.10)	0.52	1.6	3.9	7.6	14.5
	3	–	–	0.42	1.4	3.3	6.6	13.0
	4	–	–	0.29	1.1	2.6	5.2	11.0
	5	–	–	0.21	0.85	2.0	4.4	8.6
	6	–	–	0.16	(0.67)	1.7	3.8	7.5
	8	–	–	0.10	(0.48)	(1.3)	2.8	5.6
	10	–	–	–	(0.34)	(1.0)	(2.3)	4.6
	0.1	(0.74)	(1.2)	(2.1)	(3.7)	(6.9)	–	–
	0.2	0.37	0.70	(1.8)	(2.9)	(5.5)	(9.4)	(19)
	0.3	0.25	0.47	1.2	2.3	(5.0)	(8.0)	(15)
	0.4	0.17	0.36	1.0	2.0	(4.5)	(7.4)	(14)
	0.5	0.14	0.28	0.86	1.9	4.0	7.0	(13)
	0.6	0.11	0.24	0.74	1.6	3.5	6.6	12
	0.8	0.07	0.17	0.63	1.5	3.1	6.0	10
80 cm	1	0.05	0.14	0.53	1.3	2.8	5.5	9.4
	1.5	–	0.08	0.35	0.94	2.1	4.5	7.4
	2	–	(0.05)	0.26	0.74	1.8	3.5	6.2
	2.5	–	(0.04)	0.21	0.63	1.5	3.0	5.7
	3	–	–	0.16	0.55	1.3	2.6	5.2
	4	–	–	0.11	0.43	1.0	2.1	4.3
	5	–	–	0.08	0.33	0.80	1.7	3.4
	6	–	–	0.06	(0.26)	0.66	1.5	3.0
	8	–	–	0.04	(0.19)	(0.50)	1.1	2.2
	10	–	–	–	(0.13)	(0.40)	(0.9)	1.8

Mean energy and dose rate of X-rays for various filtrations (approximate values)
Mittlere Energie und Dosisleistung von Röntgenstrahlen bei verschiedener Filterung (Richtwerte)
Energie moyenne et débit de dose des rayons X pour différentes filtrations (valeurs moyennes)
Energía promedio e índice de dosis de rayos-X para diferentes filtraciones (valores aproximados)

Mean energy/peak energy – Mittlere Energie/Grenzenergie
Energie moyenne/énergie maximale – Energía promedio/energía pico

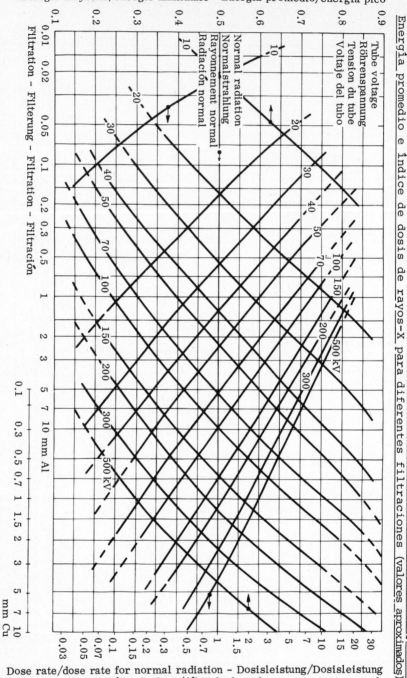

Tube voltage
Röhrenspannung
Tension du tube
Voltaje del tubo

Normal radiation
Normalstrahlung
Rayonnement normal
Radiación normal

Filtration – Filterung – Filtration – Filtración

Dose rate/dose rate for normal radiation – Dosisleistung/Dosisleistung
Normalstrahlung – Débit de dose/débit de dose du rayonnement normal –
Indice de dosis/indice de dosis para radiación normal

See pages – Siehe Seiten – Voir pages – Ver páginas 68 – 69, 74 – 77

3.6   Conversion of pulsed voltages into constant potential
      Umrechnung von pulsierenden Spannungen in Gleichspannung
      Conversion de tension pulsée en tension constante
      Conversión de voltaje pulsatil a voltaje constante

Pulsed voltages (kV~ and kV≋) required to produce radiation approximately equivalent with respect to HVL and exposure rate to radiation from an X-ray tube operated with constant potential (kV=).

Pulsierende Spannungen (kV~ und kV≋), die eingestellt werden müssen, um bezüglich HWSD und Dosisleistung einer mit Gleichspannung (kV=) betriebenen Röntgenröhre etwa äquivalente Strahlungen zu erhalten.

Tensions pulsées (kV~ et kV≋) produisant des rayonnements équivalents à celui fourni par une tension constante (kV=) en ce qui concerne la CDA et le débit d'exposition.

Voltajes pulsantes de tubo (kV~ y kV≋) para obtener radiaciones aproximadamente equivalentes en relación de CHR y exposición a las obtenidas por un tubo que opere con potencial constante (kV=).

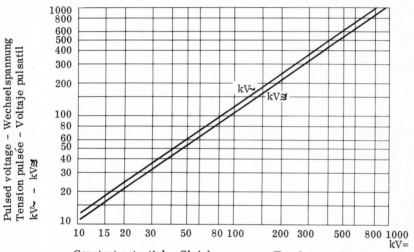

Constant potential - Gleichspannung - Tension constante
Voltaje constante

Equivalent tube voltages - Äquivalente Röhrenspannungen - Tensions équivalentes - Voltajes equivalentes en el tubo											
kV=	kV~	kV≋	kV=	kV~	kV≋	kV=	kV~	kV≋	kV=	kV~	kV≋
10	12	10.5	40	49	42	90	110	95	300	365	315
15	18	16	50	61	53	100	122	105	400	490	420
20	24	21	60	73	63	150	183	157	500	610	525
25	30	26	70	85	74	200	244	210	700	850	735
30	37	32	80	98	84	250	305	262	1000	1220	1050

Lit.: 1. Mc CULLOUGH, E.C., CAMERON, J.R.:Brit.J.Radiol.43,448(1970)
      2. KELLEY, J.P., TROUT, D.E.: Radiation Physics 100,653(1971)
      3. Authors' measurements - Eigene Messungen - Mesures
         personnelles - Medidas propias

3.7 Attenuation of X-rays in air
Schwächung von Röntgenstrahlen in Luft
Atténuation des rayons X dans l'air
Atenuación de los rayos X en el aire

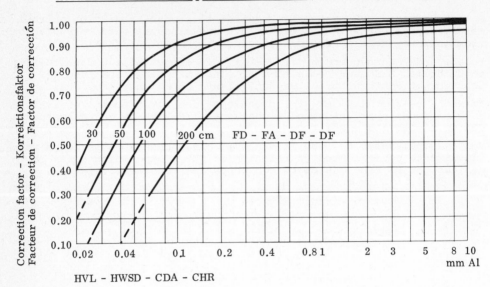

HVL - HWSD - CDA - CHR

Correction factor for the exposure calculated according to the inverse square low from the exposure at 10 cm FD - Korrektionsfaktor für die aus der Dosis in 10 cm FA nach dem Quadratgesetz berechneten Dosis - Facteur de correction de l'exposition calculée par l'inverse carré des distances à partir d'une DF de 10 cm - Factor de corrección de la exposición calculada conforme la ley del cuadrado para la exposición a partir de 10 cm DF

HVL-HWSD-CDA-CHR mm Al	FD - FA - DF - DF			cm
	30	50	100	200
0.02	0.40	0.20	–	–
0.03	0.62	0.41	0.21	–
0.05	0.80	0.65	0.45	(0.20)
0.07	0.87	0.74	0.59	0.33
0.1	0.91	0.82	0.70	0.45
0.15	0.94	0.88	0.78	0.59
0.2	0.96	0.92	0.82	0.67
0.3	0.97	0.93	0.87	0.75
0.5	0.98	0.94	0.91	0.82
0.7	0.98	0.96	0.93	0.87
1.0	0.99	0.97	0.95	0.90
1.5	0.99	0.97	0.96	0.91
2.0	0.99	0.98	0.96	0.92
3.0	1.00	0.99	0.97	0.94
5.0	1.00	0.99	0.98	0.96
10.0	1.00	1.00	0.99	0.97

Lit.: 1. WACHSMANN, F.: Hdb. Haut- und Geschlechtskrankheiten, Ergänzungsband V/2, Berlin: Springer 1959
2. See page 61 - Siehe Seite 62 - Voir page 63 - Ver página 64

3.8 <u>Examples of X-ray spectra (narrow beam)</u>
     <u>Beispiele von Röntgenspektren (enges Bündel)</u>
     <u>Exemples de spectres de rayons X (faisceaux étroits)</u>
     <u>Ejemplos de espectros de rayos-X (haz estrecho)</u>

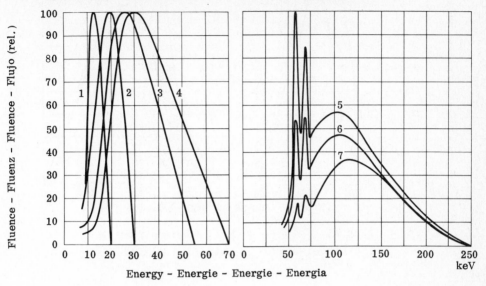

Energy - Energie - Energie - Energia

1. 20 kV=; 0.14 mm Al *)
2. 30 kV=; 0.3 mm Al
3. 55 kV=; 0.8 mm Al
4. 70 kV=; 1.25 mm Al

5. 250 kV=; 1.5 mm Cu *)
6. 250 kV=; 2.0 mm Cu
7. 250 kV=; 2.7 mm Cu

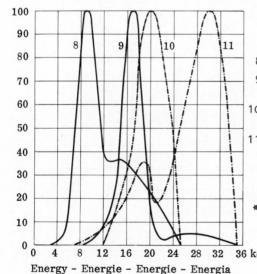

8. W-Anode; 25 kV= 1 mm Be*)

9. Idem behind - hinter -
   après - detras 8 cm H_2O

10. Mo Anode; 35 kV=
    0.05 mm Mo *)

11. Idem behind - hinter -
    après - detras 8 cm H_2O

*) Filtration - Filterung
   Filtration - Filtración

Energy - Energie - Energie - Energia

Lit.: 1. PEAPLE, L.H.J., BURT, A.K.: Phys.Med.Biol. <u>11</u>, 225 (1966)
      2. DREXLER, G.: Proceedings of the XIII Intern. Congress of
         Rad. Madrid 1973, International Congress Series No. 339,
         Excerpta Medica, Amsterdam

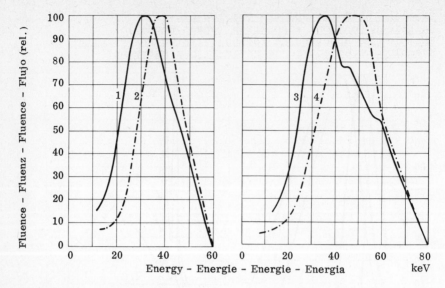

1. 60 kV=; 2 mm Al

2. Idem behind-hinter-après-
   detras 20 cm H_2O **)

3. 80 kV=; 2 mm Al

4. Idem behind-hinter-après-
   detras 20 cm H_2O **)

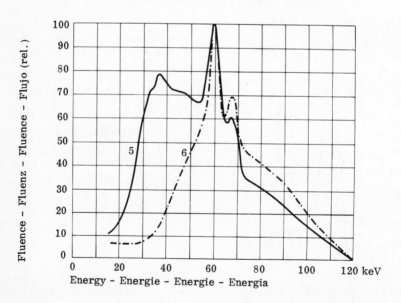

5. 120 kV=; 2 mm Al

6. Idem behind - hinter - après -
   detras 20 cm H_2O **)

**) Spectra 1-6 show clearly that, in X-ray diagnosis, only the ener-
getic radiation reaches the image recorder, and that low-energy components only cause unnecessary exposure to the patient.

Die Spektren 1-6 zeigen deutlich, daß in der Röntgendiagnostik
nur die energiereichen Anteile bis zum Bildempfänger gelangen
und daß die weichen den Patienten nur unnötig belasten.

**) Les spectres no 1-6 montrent clairement qu'en radiodiagnostic
     seuls les rayonnements des plus hautes énergies atteignent
     le detecteur tandis que les rayonnements de plus faible énergie
     ne font que délivrer une dose inutile au malade.

     Los esprectros muestran claramente que en el radiodiagnostico
     solamente los rayos energéticos alcanzan el detector de imagen
     y que los blandos solo cargan inutilmente al paciente.

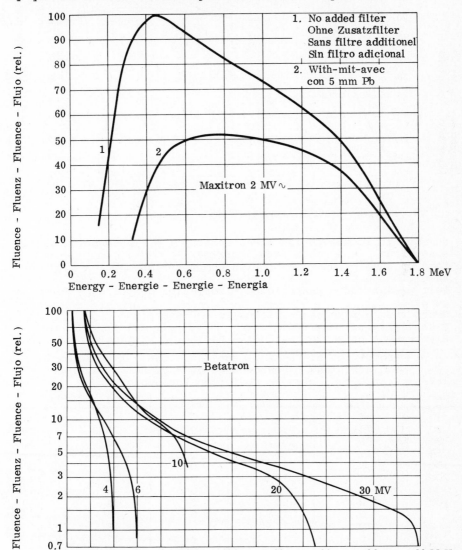

Lit.: 1. SAYLOR, W.L.: Phys.Med.Biol. 14, 87 (1969)
      2. MARUYAMA, T., SAKATA, S., KUMAMOTO, Y., HASHIZUME, T.,
         HATTORI, H., KANAMORI, H., YAMAMOTO, M.: Health Phys. 28,
         777 (1975)

3.9 Attenuation processes of X rays in a 10 cm layer of water
Schwächungsprozesse von Röntgenstrahlung in 10 cm Wasser
Modes d'atténuation des rayons X dans 10 cm d'eau
Procesos por disminuir los rayos X en 10 cm de agua

100 cm^2 Field size - Feld - Champ - Campo

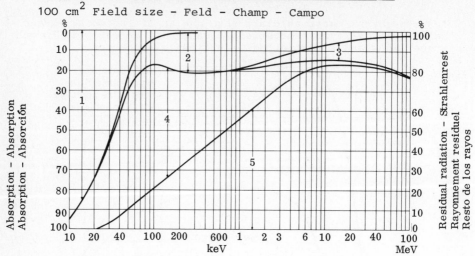

Energie - Energy - Energie - Energía

1. Photoelectric absorption - Photoabsorption - Absorption photoélectrique - Absorción fotoeléctrica
2. Compton absorption - Absorption compton - Absorption compton -
   Absorción compton
3. Pair production - Paarbildung - Formation de paires - Formación
   de pares
4. Scattering - Streuung - Diffusion - Dispersión
5. Transmitted primary radiation - Unbeeinflußter Strahlenrest -
   Rayonnement primaire résiduel - Radiación residual inalterada

E keV/ MeV	Proportion of the incident radiation - Anteile an der Ein- fallstrahlung - Pourcentage du rayonnement incident - Participación en la radiación incidente %				
	1	2	3	4	5
10	95	0	0	5	∿0
20	75	∿0	0	25	∿0
30	55	2.5	0	40	2.5
50	21	9	0	60	10
100	4.0	13	0	63	20
200	1.0	19	0	48	32
300	0	20	0	42	38
500	0	20	0	34	46
1	0	18	0	25	57
2	0	14	3	16	67
3	0	12	4	11	73
5	0	9.5	5.5	6.5	79
10	0	6.0	7.5	2.5	84
20	0	4.0	10	2.0	84
30	0	2.0	12	2.0	84
50	0	2.0	15	1.0	82
70	0	1.2	18	0.8	80
100	0	1.0	21	∿0	78

Table of contents - Inhaltsverzeichnis
Table des matières - Tabla de materias

4.1 Central axis relative depth doses for X-rays
Relative Tiefendosen im Zentralstrahl für Röntgenstrahlen
Rendements relatives en profondeur sur l'axe pour les rayons X
Dosis relativas en profundidad en el eje central para rayos X

General information - Allgemeine Erklärungen - Explications
générales - Explicaciónes generales

The values given on the following pages for the "relative depth doses" based on the surface or maximum dose are for the quality of radiation (HVL), focus-skin distance (FSD), and field size (cm^2) indicated, for measurements in "infinite" phantoms. The numbers in the
tables are rounded off, since more precise values are uncertain and
of no practical significance. Unreliable data are indicated in the
graphs by dashed lines, and in the tables, by parentheses.

Die auf den folgenden Seiten angegebenen Werte für die auf die Ober-
flächen- bzw. Maximaldosen bezogenen "relativen Tiefendosen" gelten
für die jeweils angegebenen Strahlenqualitäten (HWSD), Fokus-Hautab-
stände (FHA) und Feldgrößen (cm^2) für Messungen in "unendlich großen"
Phantomen. In den Tabellen sind abgerundete Zahlen angegeben, da ge-
nauere Werte unsicher und für die Praxis ohne Bedeutung sind. Nicht
zuverlässige Angaben sind in den Kurven gestrichelt und in den Tabellen eingeklammert angegeben.

Les valeurs données dans les pages suivantes pour les "rendements
relatifs en profondeur" sont rapportées à la dose à la surface ou
à la dose maximale, pour différentes qualités de rayonnement (CDA),
distances foyer-peau (DFP) et dimensions de champ (cm^2) et correspon-
dent à des mesures dans un fantôme "semi-infini". Les valeurs données dans les tables sont arrondies car le chiffre suivant serait
imprécis et sans signification pratique. Les valeurs qui ne sont pas
sûres sont mises entre parenthèses dans les tables et sont represen-
tées par des courbes pointillées dans les figures.

Los valores de las "dosis en profundidad relativas" referidas a la
dosis superficial o máxima, que se indican en las páginas se refie-
ren a la calidad de la radiación (CHR), distancia foco-piel (DFP) y
amplitud de campo (cm^2) para medidas en fantomas de "tamano infini-
to". Los números que figuran en las tablas estan redondeados a ya
que valores más exactos son inseguros y carecen de importancia práctica. Los datos que no son de total confianza aparecen plumeados en
las curvas y entre parêntesis en las tablas.

Lit.: 1. IAEA, Atlas of Radiation Dose Distribution, Vol. 1, Vienna
         1965
      2. RUDERMAN, A.J., BIBEGAL, A.A., VAINBERG, M.Sh.: Atlas of
         Dose Fields, 1, SSSR: Moscow 1968
      3. JOHNS, H.E., CUNNINGHAM, J.R.: The Physics of Radiology,
         3th Edit., Springfield: C.C.Thomas 1969
      4. Brit.J.Radiol., Suppl. 11, London 1972
      5. Authors' measurements - Eigene Messungen - Mesures person-
         nelles - Medidas propias

These references also apply to pages - Diese Literaturstellen gelten
auch für die Seiten - Ces références se rapportent aussi aux pages -
Estas indicaciones bibliográficas valen también para las páginas
87, 104, 118, 126, 128.

4.2 Low energy X-rays - Weiche Röntgenstrahlen - Rayons X mous - Rayos X blandos

4.2.1 0.02 - 0.8 mm Al HVL - HWSD - CDA - CHR

(10) - 30 - (50) cm FSD - FHA - DFP - DFP

(10) - 100 - (400) cm^2 Field size - Feldgröße - Champ - Campo

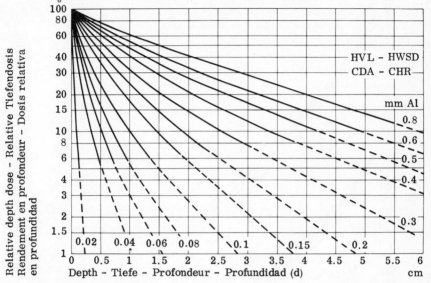

d	Depth doses - Tiefendosen - Rendement en profondeur - Dosis en profundidad							%
cm	HVL - HWSD - CDA - CHR: mm Al				d			
	0.02	0.04	0.06	0.08	cm	0.04	0.06	0.08
0.02	50	76	86	78	0.4	(7.8)	14.5	21
0.04	30	66	72	90	0.5	(5.4)	10.5	16.5
0.06	20	52	62	67	0.6	(4.0)	(7.8)	13.5
0.08	13	46	59	66	0.8	(2.1)	(4.6)	(8.0)
0.10	(9)	38	54	62	1.0	(1.1)	(3.0)	(5.5)
0.15	(3.7)	27	36	45	1.2	–	(2.0)	(4.0)
0.20	(1.5)	20	33	41	1.4	–	(1.5)	(2.8)
0.25	–	15.0	26	34	1.6	–	(< 1)	(2.0)
0.30	–	12.0	21	29	1.8	–	–	(1.5)

d cm	0.1	0.15	0.2	0.3	0.4	0.5	0.6	0.8
0.1	62	78	81	85	88	92	95	97
0.2	50	62	68	76	80	84	88	91
0.4	30	43	49	59	66	72	77	82
0.6	20	31	38	48	56	62	68	75
0.8	14.5	24	29	39	48	54	60	68
1	10.0	17.5	24	32	41	48	54	62
1.5	(5.0)	9.7	14.5	21	29	36	42	50
2	(2.7)	(5.6)	(9.0)	14.5	21	27	33	41
2.5	(1.6)	(3.4)	(6.5)	10.5	16.0	21	26	35
3	(< 1)	(2.1)	(4.1)	(7.6)	12.0	17.0	22	29
4	–	–	(1.9)	(4.2)	(7.5)	11.5	14.5	20
5	–	–	(< 1)	(2.4)	(4.8)	(7.0)	9.6	14.0

<u>1 mm Al HVL - HWSD - CDA - CHR</u>
15 - 30 - 50 cm FSD - FHA - DFP - DFP
10 - 400 cm^2 Field size - Feldgröße - Champ - Campo

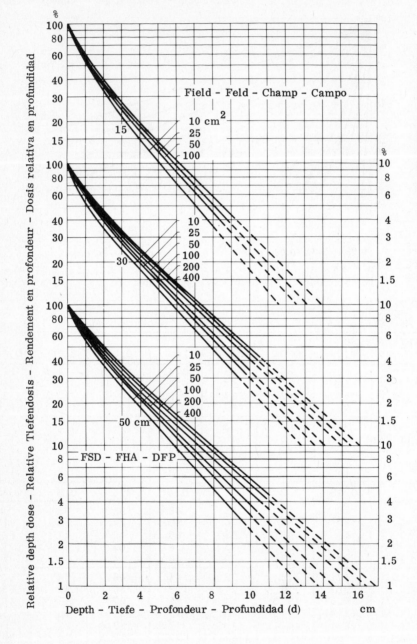

FSD FHA DFP	d cm	Field size - Feldgröße - Champ - Campo:					cm^2
		10	25	50	100	200	400
15 cm	0	100	100	100	100		
	0.5	65	68	70	73		
	1	53	55	57	60		
	1.5	40	44	46	50		
	2	32	35	37	40		
	3	21	24	26	28		
	4	15.0	17.0	18.5	20		
	5	10.5	12.5	13.5	14.5		
	6	7.3	8.8	9.4	11.0		
	7	5.2	6.3	7	7.8		
	8	3.6	4.6	5.1	5.8		
	9	2.5	3.2	(3.6)	(4.3)		
	10	1.8	(2.3)	(2.7)	(3.2)		
	11	(1.2)	(1.7)	(2.0)	(2.4)		
	12	–	(1.4)	(1.5)	(1.8)		
	13	–	–	(1.0)	(1.3)		
30 cm	0	100	100	100	100	100	100
	0.5	65	71	75	77	79	81
	1	53	60	62	64	67	70
	1.5	44	50	52	55	56	58
	2	35	39	41	43	45	46
	3	25	27	29	31	33	34
	4	18.0	19.5	21	23	24	25
	5	13.5	14.5	15.5	16.5	18.0	18.5
	6	9.2	10.5	11.5	12.5	13.5	14.0
	7	6.8	7.8	8.3	9.6	10.5	11.5
	8	4.8	5.7	6.3	7.3	7.9	8.4
	9	3.5	4.2	4.7	5.6	6.1	6.4
	10	(2.5)	(3.0)	(3.5)	4.2	4.5	5.0
	11	(1.8)	(2.2)	(2.6)	(3.1)	(3.4)	(3.7)
	12	(1.4)	(1.7)	(1.9)	(2.4)	(2.7)	(2.9)
	13	–	(1.2)	(1.4)	(1.7)	(2.0)	(2.2)
	14	–	–	(1.0)	(1.3)	(1.5)	(1.7)
	15	–	–	–	(1.0)	(1.2)	(1.3)
	16	–	–	–	–	–	(1.1)
50 cm	0	100	100	100	100	100	100
	0.5	70	74	76	78	80	82
	1	56	60	63	66	68	70
	1.5	46	49	51	54	56	58
	2	38	42	44	46	48	50
	3	18.5	29	41	43	45	47
	4	13.5	21	23	24	26	28
	5	14	15.5	17.0	18.5	20	22
	6	9.6	11.5	12.5	14.0	15.5	16.5
	7	7.0	8.4	9.4	10.5	12.0	13.0
	8	5.0	6.0	7.0	8.2	9.2	10.0
	9	3.6	4.5	5.2	6.2	7.1	7.7
	10	(2.6)	3.2	3.9	4.8	5.4	6.0
	11	(1.8)	(2.4)	(2.9)	(3.6)	4.2	4.6
	12	(1.4)	(1.8)	(2.2)	(2.8)	(3.2)	(3.6)
	13	(1.0)	(1.2)	(1.6)	(2.1)	(2.4)	(2.7)
	14	–	–	–	(1.6)	(1.9)	(2.1)
	15	–	–	–	(1.2)	(1.4)	(1.6)
	16	–	–	–	–	(1.1)	(1.3)

2 mm Al HVL – HWSD – CDA – CHR
15 – 30 – 50 cm FSD – FHA – DFP – DFP
10 – 400 cm^2 Field size – Feldgröße – Champ – Campo

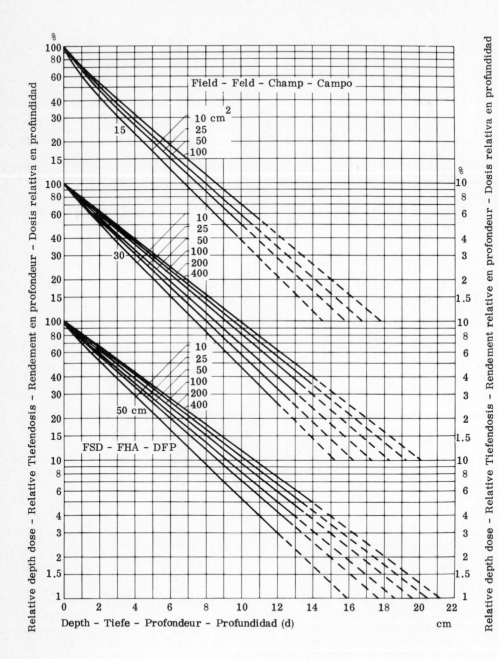

FSD FHA DFP	d cm	Field size - Feldgröße - Champ - Campo:					cm²
		10	25	50	100	200	400
15 cm	0.5	76	80	82	84		
	1	60	68	70	73		
	1.5	50	58	60	63		
	2	42	48	50	54		
	3	32	37	39	43		
	4	23	27	29	32		
	5	17.5	20	22	25		
	6	12.5	15.0	17.0	19.0		
	7	9.4	12.0	13.5	15.0		
	8	6.4	8.6	9.8	11.5		
	9	5.2	6.6	7.6	9.0		
	10	(3.8)	4.0	5.8	6.9		
	12	(2.2)	(2.9)	(3.5)	(4.3)		
	14	(1.2)	(1.5)	(2.0)	(2.5)		
	16	–	–	(1.4)	(1.5)		
	18	–	–	–	(1.0)		
30 cm	0.5	84	87	88	89	90	91
	1	70	74	76	78	79	80
	1.5	60	64	66	68	70	72
	2	50	55	57	60	63	65
	3	37	41	43	46	48	50
	4	27	30	33	36	38	39
	5	20	23	25	28	30	32
	6	15.0	17.5	19.5	22	23	25
	7	11.5	13.5	15.0	17.0	18.5	19.5
	8	8.4	10.0	11.5	13.5	14.5	15.5
	9	6.2	7.6	8.9	10.5	11.5	12.5
	10	4.6	5.7	6.8	8.2	9.0	10.0
	12	2.6	3.3	4.0	5.0	5.6	6.3
	14	(1.4)	(1.9)	(2.4)	(2.9)	3.5	4.0
	16	–	(1.1)	(1.4)	(1.8)	(2.2)	(2.5)
	18	–	–	–	(1.1)	(1.3)	(1.6)
	20	–	–	–	–	–	(1.0)
50 cm	0.5	79	83	87	89	91	93
	1	69	74	75	77	81	83
	1.5	59	64	66	68	72	73
	2	52	57	60	62	65	67
	3	38	43	45	48	52	54
	4	29	33	35	38	41	44
	5	22	26	28	31	33	35
	6	16.5	20	22	24	26	28
	7	12.5	15.5	17.0	19.0	21	22
	8	9.2	12.5	13.5	15.0	16.5	18.5
	9	7.0	9.1	10.5	12.0	13.5	14.5
	10	5.2	7.1	8.1	9.8	11.0	12.0
	12	3.0	4.2	5.0	6.0	6.7	7.6
	14	(1.7)	(2.5)	(3.2)	(3.7)	(4.3)	5.9
	16	(1.0)	(1.5)	(1.9)	(2.3)	(2.7)	(3.1)
	18	–	–	(1.1)	(1.4)	(1.7)	(2.0)
	20	–	–	–	–	(1.1)	(1.3)

4.2.4 3 mm Al HVL – HWSD – CDA – CHR
15 – 30 – 50 cm FSD – FHA – DFP – DFP
10 – 400 cm^2 Field size – Feldgröße – Champ – Campo

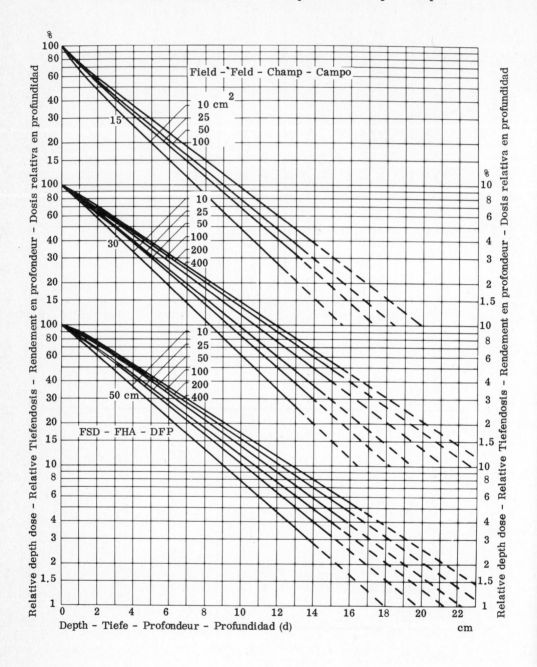

FSD FHA DFP	d cm	Field size - Feldgröße - Champ - Campo:					cm^2
		10	25	50	100	200	400
15 cm	0.5	80	82	84	86		
	1	66	72	74	76		
	1.5	56	62	64	66		
	2	47	54	56	58		
	3	35	41	43	47		
	4	26	31	33	36		
	5	19.5	24	26	29		
	6	15.0	19.0	20	24		
	7	12.5	15.0	16.5	18.5		
	8	8.3	11.5	12.5	15.0		
	9	6.4	8.7	9.8	12.0		
	10	4.8	6.7	7.7	9.5		
	12	2.7	4.0	4.7	6.1		
	14	(1.5)	(2.3)	(2.9)	(3.7)		
	16	-	(1.4)	(1.7)	(2.4)		
	18	-	-	(1.1)	(1.5)		
	20	-	-	-	(1.0)		
30 cm	0.5	87	89	90	92	93	94
	1	76	79	81	84	85	87
	1.5	65	68	70	72	74	76
	2	57	61	63	66	68	70
	3	44	49	51	54	56	58
	4	33	37	39	43	45	46
	5	25	29	31	34	36	38
	6	19.0	23	25	28	30	32
	7	14.0	18.0	20	23	25	27
	8	11.0	13.5	15.5	18.0	20	21
	9	8.0	11.5	12.0	14.5	16.5	17.5
	10	6.1	8.2	9.7	12.0	13.5	14.5
	12	3.5	5.0	6.0	7.8	9.0	10.0
	14	(2.0)	(3.0)	(3.7)	4.9	6.0	6.7
	16	(1.1)	(1.7)	(2.2)	(3.0)	(3.9)	4.4
	18	-	(1.0)	(1.4)	(2.0)	(2.6)	(3.0)
	20	-	-	-	(1.3)	(1.8)	(2.1)
	22	-	-	-	-	(1.2)	(1.4)
50 cm	0.5	88	92	93	95	96	97
	1	78	83	85	88	90	91
	1.5	68	74	75	78	81	83
	2	60	65	68	72	74	76
	3	47	53	55	60	62	64
	4	36	42	44	48	50	52
	5	28	33	35	40	41	43
	6	22	26	28	33	35	36
	7	17.0	21	23	26	28	30
	8	13.0	16.5	18.5	21	23	25
	9	10.0	13.5	15.0	17.5	19.0	21
	10	7.6	10.5	12.0	14.0	15.5	17.0
	12	4.6	6.3	7.5	9.0	10.5	12.0
	14	2.8	3.9	4.9	5.8	7.0	8.0
	16	(1.6)	(2.4)	(3.0)	3.7	4.6	5.4
	18	(1.0)	(1.5)	(2.0)	(2.4)	(3.1)	(3.7)
	20	-	(1.0)	(1.3)	(1.6)	(2.0)	(2.5)
	22	-	-	-	(1.0)	(1.4)	(1.7)

4.2.5   <u>4 mm Al HVL - HWSD - CDA - CHR</u>
        15 - 30 - 50 cm FSD - FHA - DFP - DFP
        10 - 400 cm^2 Field size - Feldgröße - Champ - Campo

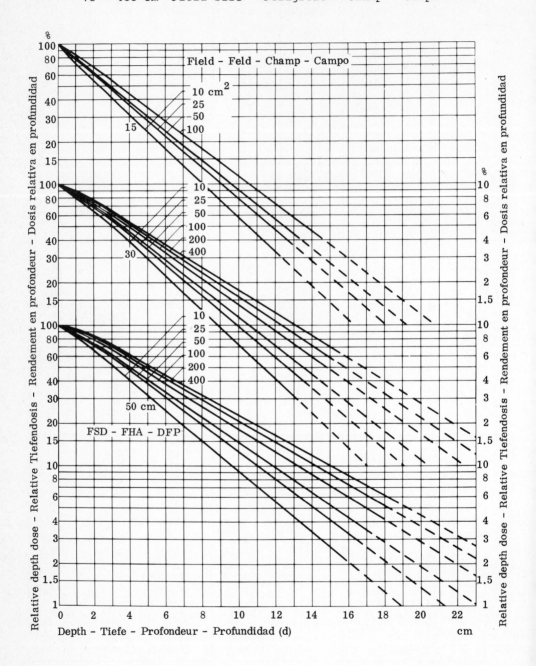

Field - Feld - Champ - Campo

Depth - Tiefe - Profondeur - Profundidad (d)   cm

Relative depth dose - Relative Tiefendosis - Rendement en profondeur - Dosis relativa en profundidad

FSD FHA DFP	d cm	Field size - Feldgröße - Champ - Campo:					cm²
		10	25	50	100	200	400
15 cm	0.5	84	87	89	92		
	1	72	76	78	84		
	1.5	63	68	70	76		
	2	54	60	62	68		
	3	41	46	48	54		
	4	31	36	38	44		
	5	24	28	30	35		
	6	17.5	22	24	28		
	7	13.5	17.0	19.0	22		
	8	10.5	13.0	15.0	18.0		
	9	7.7	10.0	11.5	14.5		
	10	5.8	7.8	9.0	11.5		
	12	3.4	4.8	5.8	7.3		
	14	(1.9)	(2.8)	(3.5)	4.6		
	16	(1.1)	(1.7)	(2.2)	(2.9)		
	18	-	(1.0)	(1.3)	(1.9)		
	20	-	-	-	(1.2)		
30 cm	0.5	89	91	93	95	96	97
	1	79	82	84	86	88	90
	1.5	71	75	77	78	79	83
	2	64	69	70	74	75	77
	3	50	54	57	60	62	64
	4	38	43	46	49	52	54
	5	29	34	36	39	42	44
	6	22	27	29	32	35	37
	7	17.0	21	23	26	29	31
	8	13.0	16.5	17.5	21	23	25
	9	9.6	12.5	14.5	17.5	19.5	22
	10	7.2	9.8	11.5	14.0	16.0	18.0
	12	4.1	5.8	7.1	9.0	10.5	12.0
	14	(2.4)	3.6	4.5	6.0	7.2	8.6
	16	(1.3)	(2.1)	(2.8)	3.8	4.7	5.8
	18	-	(1.3)	(1.7)	(2.6)	(3.3)	(4.0)
	20	-	-	(1.1)	(1.7)	(2.2)	(2.8)
	22	-	-	-	(1.1)	(1.5)	(1.9)
50 cm	0.5	91	93	94	96	97	98
	1	83	87	89	92	94	96
	1.5	74	78	82	85	88	90
	2	66	71	73	77	81	84
	3	52	58	62	66	70	73
	4	40	48	50	56	59	62
	5	32	38	41	46	49	52
	6	25	30	33	38	42	44
	7	19.5	25	28	32	35	38
	8	15.0	20.0	22	26	29	32
	9	12.5	16.0	18.0	23	26	28
	10	9.4	12.5	14.5	18.5	21	23
	12	5.4	8.0	9.7	12.5	15.0	17.0
	14	3.5	5.2	6.7	8.6	10.5	12.0
	16	(2.1)	(3.4)	(4.4)	6.0	7.4	8.6
	18	(1.2)	(2.1)	(2.8)	(4.2)	5.2	6.2
	20	-	(1.3)	(1.8)	(2.8)	(3.6)	(4.4)
	22	-	-	(1.3)	(2.0)	(2.6)	(3.2)

4.2.6 <u>6 mm Al HVL - HWSD - CDA - CHR</u>

15 - 30 - 50 cm FSD - FHA - DFP - DFP

10 - 400 cm^2 Field size - Feldgröße - Champ - Campo

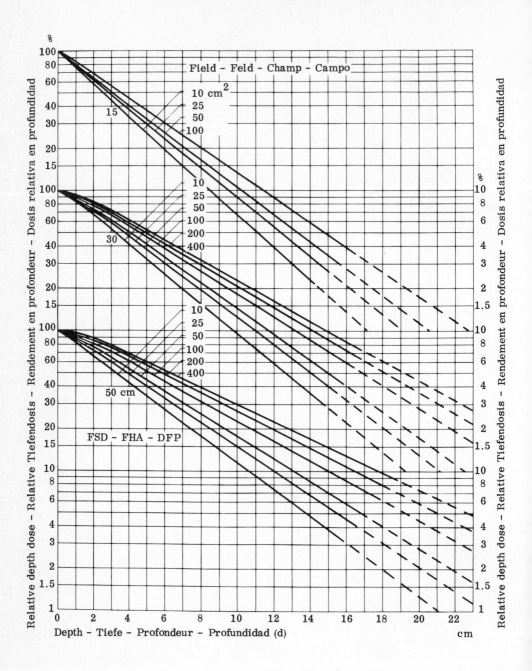

FSD FHA DFP	d cm	Field size - Feldgröße - Champ - Campo: 10	25	50	100	200	cm² 400
15 cm	0.5	87	88	90	93		
	1	76	78	80	83		
	1.5	66	69	72	76		
	2	58	62	64	69		
	3	44	48	50	56		
	4	34	38	40	46		
	5	26	30	33	38		
	6	19.5	24	26	31		
	7	15.0	18.5	21	25		
	8	11.0	14.5	16.5	20		
	9	8.8	11.0	13.0	16.5		
	10	6.7	9.0	10.5	13.0		
	12	4.0	5.6	6.8	9.0		
	14	(2.3)	(3.4)	(4.3)	6.0		
	16	(1.4)	(2.1)	(2.8)	(4.0)		
	18	-	(1.3)	(1.8)	(2.7)		
	20	-	-	(1.1)	(1.7)		
	22	-	-	-	(1.2)		
30 cm	0.5	90	92	93	95	97	98
	1	83	86	88	91	93	96
	1.5	75	78	81	84	86	88
	2	66	70	73	77	80	83
	3	52	58	61	66	70	73
	4	42	48	51	56	59	62
	5	32	38	42	47	50	53
	6	25	31	34	39	42	45
	7	20	25	28	33	36	38
	8	15.5	19.5	22	27	29	32
	9	12.0	15.5	18.5	23	25	27
	10	9.5	12.5	14.5	18.0	21	23
	12	6.0	8.2	9.7	12.5	15.0	16.5
	14	3.7	5.2	6.4	8.8	10.0	11.5
	16	(2.2)	3.2	4.1	6.0	7.3	8.6
	18	(1.4)	(2.0)	(3.6)	(4.1)	(5.1)	(6.1)
	20	-	(1.3)	(1.8)	(2.8)	(3.6)	(4.4)
	22	-	-	(1.1)	(1.9)	(2.6)	(3.1)
50 cm	0.5	92	94	96	97	98	99
	1	84	89	90	93	96	98
	1.5	74	80	82	86	90	96
	2	67	74	78	82	86	90
	3	52	60	64	70	74	78
	4	43	49	54	61	66	70
	5	35	40	45	52	57	60
	6	28	33	37	44	50	53
	7	22	27	31	33	43	46
	8	17.5	22	25	31	36	39
	9	14.0	18.0	21	27	31	34
	10	11.5	15.0	17.5	23	27	30
	12	7.4	10.0	12.0	16.0	20	23
	14	4.8	6.7	8.5	11.5	14.5	17.0
	16	(3.0)	(4.5)	5.8	8.4	10.5	12.5
	18	(1.9)	(3.0)	(4.0)	(6.1)	(7.8)	9.7
	20	(1.2)	(2.0)	(2.8)	(4.5)	(5.8)	(7.3)
	22	-	(1.4)	(1.9)	(3.2)	(4.3)	(5.2)

4.2.7   <u>8 mm Al HVL - HWSD - CDA - CHR</u>
<u>15 - 30 - 50 cm FSD - FHA - DFP - DFP</u>
<u>10 - 400 cm^2 Field size - Feldgröße - Champ - Campo</u>

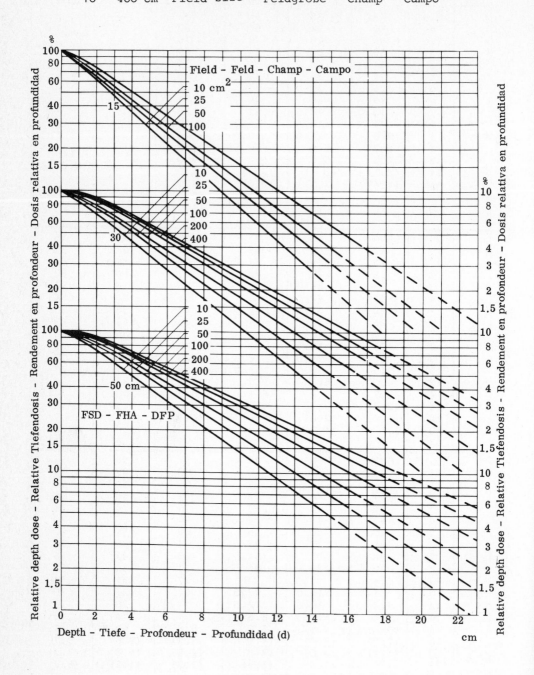

Field - Feld - Champ - Campo

10 cm^2
25
50
100

FSD - FHA - DFP

Relative depth dose - Relative Tiefendosis - Rendement en profondeur - Dosis relativa en profundidad

Depth - Tiefe - Profondeur - Profundidad (d)   cm

FSD FHA DFP	d cm	Field size − Feldgröße − Champ − Campo:					cm²
		10	25	50	100	200	400
15 cm	0.5	90	92	94	97		
	1	79	82	84	89		
	1.5	70	73	76	82		
	2	62	66	70	76		
	3	47	51	55	62		
	4	36	40	45	50		
	5	28	32	35	42		
	6	22	25	28	34		
	7	16.5	20	23	28		
	8	13.0	16.0	18.5	23		
	9	9.7	12.5	15.0	19.0		
	10	7.7	9.8	11.5	15.5		
	12	4.6	6.2	7.8	10.5		
	14	(2.7)	3.8	4.9	7.0		
	16	(1.6)	(2.4)	(3.2)	4.7		
	18	−	(1.5)	(2.0)	(3.0)		
	20	−	−	(1.3)	(2.1)		
	22	−	−	−	(1.4)		
30 cm	0.5	90	94	95	97	98	99
	1	83	88	90	93	95	97
	1.5	77	83	86	90	93	95
	2	68	75	78	84	87	90
	3	54	61	66	72	75	78
	4	44	51	55	62	66	68
	5	36	40	45	52	55	58
	6	27	33	37	44	47	50
	7	22	27	32	37	40	43
	8	17.0	22	26	30	34	37
	9	13.5	17.5	21	26	28	31
	10	10.5	14.0	17.0	21	24	26
	12	6.6	9.4	12.0	15.0	17.0	19.5
	14	4.2	6.2	8.2	10.5	12.0	14.0
	16	(2.5)	(4.0)	5.5	7.5	8.7	10.0
	18	(1.6)	(2.6)	(3.6)	(5.2)	(6.2)	7.5
	20	(1.0)	(1.7)	(2.5)	(3.8)	(4.5)	(5.5)
	22	−	(1.1)	(1.7)	(2.6)	(3.3)	(4.0)
50 cm	0.5	93	95	96	98	99	100
	1	88	93	94	96	97	98
	1.5	80	86	88	92	94	96
	2	73	80	83	88	90	92
	3	60	68	72	78	80	82
	4	49	56	62	67	70	73
	5	40	47	52	57	60	63
	6	32	38	43	49	52	55
	7	26	32	36	42	45	48
	8	21	26	30	35	40	42
	9	17.0	22	26	32	35	38
	10	14.0	18.0	21	26	30	32
	12	9.4	12.0	15.0	19.0	22	25
	14	6.1	8.3	11.0	14.0	17.0	19.0
	16	(4.0)	5.7	7.5	10.0	12.5	14.5
	18	(2.6)	(3.8)	(5.2)	(7.4)	9.2	11.0
	20	(1.8)	(2.6)	(3.7)	(5.4)	(7.0)	8.8
	22	(1.1)	(1.8)	(2.6)	(3.9)	(5.2)	(6.5)

4.2.8 Therapy with low energy X-rays, short distance- and half deep therapy
Weichstrahltherapie, Nahbestrahlung und Halbtiefentherapie
Thérapie avec rayons mous, thérapie de contact et thérapie superficielle
Terapia con rayos blandos, proximal y semiprofunda

4.2.8.1 Radiation qualities and dose rates obtained at 10 cm FSD
Strahlenqualitäten und in 10 cm FHA erreichte Dosisleistungen
Qualités de rayonnement et débits à une DFP de 10 cm
Calidad de la radiaciónes e intensidades obtenidas a 10 cm DFP

HVL - HWSD - CDA - CHR   and - und - et - y
Exposure rate-Dosisleistung-Débit d'exposition-Indice de exposición

Tube voltage - Röhrenspannung - Tension d'alimentation - Voltaje del tubo: kV=								mm Al - Cu R/min/mA
	10	20	30	40	50	60	80	100
1 mm Be	0.024 (200)	0.045 (1800)	0.050 -	0.055 -	0.057 -	0.060 -	0.065 -	0.07 -
0.1 mm Al	0.042 15	0.074 80	0.085 380	0.098 580	0.10 750	0.11 900	0.12 1150	0.13 1300
0.2 mm Al	0.06 (5)	0.11 45	0.14 150	0.15 225	0.16 340	0.17 400	0.18 530	0.21 700
0.3 mm Al	0.08 -	0.15 25	0.18 80	0.21 140	0.22 190	0.25 260	0.30 380	0.37 500
0.5 mm Al	0.13 -	0.24 12	0.32 40	0.38 80	0.42 115	0.48 155	0.62 200	0.80 320
0.8 mm Al	0.17 -	0.37 6	0.50 23	0.62 40	0.72 65	0.81 90	1.15 150	1.5 290
1.0 mm Al	0.20 -	0.45 5	0.62 17	0.80 30	0.90 48	1.00 70	1.35 130	1.70 200
1.5 mm Al	0.29 -	0.62 -	0.82 10	1.2 18	1.3 32	1.4 46	1.8 90	2.3 145
2.0 mm Al	- -	0.75 -	1.0 6.5	1.4 12	1.6 22	1.7 36	2.2 70	3.1 120
0.2 mm Cu	- -	- -	- -	- -	2.8 2.0	3.3 9.0	4.4 23	(0.2) 42
0.5 mm Cu	- -	- -	- -	- -	3.7 2.5	4.9 8.0	(0.4) 16	

(Filter - Filtre - Filtro)

Lit.: 1. OOSTERKAMP, W.J.: Acta Radiol. 33, 491 (1950)
2. CHAOUL, H., WACHSMANN, F.: Die Nahbestrahlung, Stuttgart: Thieme 1953
3. WACHSMANN, F.: Jadassohn Hdb. Haut- und Geschlechtskrankh., Band V/2, Berlin-Göttingen-Heidelberg-New York: Springer 1959
4. See pages - Siehe Seiten - Voir pages - Ver paginas 75 - 76

4.2.8.2   Approximate HVD obtained - Etwa erreichte GHWT
PDA approximative - PHR aproximadamente obtenida

HVD - GHWT - PDA - PHR   mm
with - mit - avec - con: HVL - HWSD - CDA - CHR

mm Al	0.025	0.1	0.2	0.3	0.4	0.5	0.8	1.0
1.5	0.22	-	-	-	-	-	-	-
3	0.22	0.4	0.7	1.4	1.6	1.8	-	-
5	0.22	0.6	1.2	2.4	3.0	3.2	3.5	5.0
10	0.22	1.0	2.4	3.8	4.7	6.0	7.0	9.0
15	0.22	1.4	3.0 [1]	4.8	6.2 [1]	7.6	9.5	12 [1]
20	0.22	1.7	3.5	5.4	7.0	8.7	12	14
30	0.23 [1]	2.0	4.2 [1]	6.2	8.2 [1]	10	15	17 [1]
50	0.23	2.2	4.4	6.6	8.6	10.7	16	19
100	0.23	-	-	6.7	8.8	11	17	20
200	0.23	-	-	-	-	11	17	20

(Rows labelled: FSD-FHA-DFP cm)

mm Al	1.5	2	3	4	5	6	8	10
mm Cu					0.16	0.20	0.3	0.5
1.0	-	-	-	3-4 [2]	-	-	-	-
3	-	-	-	7-9	-	-	-	-
5	8.0	13	-	10-13	-	-	-	-
10	14	20	22	26	30	35	40	42
15	18	23	27	32	35	40	43	45
20	21	24	29	35	38	43	46	48
30	23	27	33	38 [3]	42	46	50	52
50	26	29	36	43	45	50	54	57
100	27	32	41	47	48	54	58	62
200	28	34	43	50	52	56	61	65

(Rows labelled: FSD-FHA-DFP cm)

[1] Values commonly used in low-energy-therapy
In der Weichstrahltherapie häufig benützte Werte
Valeurs souvent utilisées en radiothérapie par rayons X mous
Valores generalmente usados en la terapía con rayos blandos

[2] Short distance therapy - Nahbestrahlung - Thérapie de contact -
Terapía a distancia corta (proximal)

[3] Values recommended for subcutaneous- and half deep therapy
Für die Unterhaut- und Halbtiefentherapie empfohlene Werte
Valeurs recommandées pour la radiothérapie semiprofonde
Valores recomendados para la terapía subcutánea y semiprofunda

	d		Relative depth doses - Relative Tiefendosen - Rendements en profondeur - Dosis relativa en profundidad %								
			kV and FSD - kV und FHA - kV et DFP - kV y DFP								
			Monopan			Dermopan					
			1*)	2	3	4	5	6	7	8	9
		kV	60	60	60	10	29	43	50	50	50
	cm	cm	1.5	3	5	15	15	15	15	30	200
	0.5		48	64	74	23	41	58	69	80	83
	1		31	43	48	8.8	25	39	50	68	70
	1.5		21	32	46	-	16	27	36	56	60
	2		15	23	37	-	11	20	28	46	50
	2.5		11	17	29	-	8.0	15	21	39	43
	3		8.2	13	23	-	5.8	11	17	33	36
	3.5		6.3	10	18	-	-	8.3	13	28	31
	5		-	5.0	10	-	-	-	6.4	17	19

(Left labels: I Röhren I - Siemens tubes - Tubes / Tubos)

*) 1-9 See page - Siehe Seite - Voir page - Ver página 102

4.2.8.3 Siemens Dermopan and - und - et - y Monopan

Usual operating conditions - Gebräuchliche Betriebsbe-
dingungen - Conditions normales d'utilisation - Condiciones normales de utilización

Method Methode Méthode Metodo (Therapy)	Step Stufe Reglage Grado	kV	Filter Filter Filtre Filtro mm	FSD FHA DFP DFP cm	Field Feld Champ Campo Ø cm	Dose rate Dosisleistg. Débit Intensidad R/min	Curve Kurve Courbe Curva No.
Dermopan							
Grenz rays Grenzstrahlen Rayons Bucky Rayos Grenz	I I	10∿ 10∿	∿1 Be ∿1 Be	15 30	2-4 10	∿1000/25 mA ∿1000/25 mA	1 1
Soft X-rays Weichstrahlen Rayons mous Rayos blandos	II II III III IV IV IV	29∿ 29∿ 43∿ 43∿ 50∿ 50∿ 50∿	0.3 Al 0.3 Al 0.6 Al 0.6 Al 1 Al 1 Al 1 Al	15 30 15 30 15 30 200	2-4 ∿10 2-4 ∿10 2-4 ∿10 >1000	∿400/25 mA ∿100/25 mA ∿400/25 mA ∿100/25 mA ∿400/25 mA ∿100/25 mA ∿5/25 mA	2 3 4 5 6 7 8
Monopan (Chaoul)							
Short distance or contact Nahbestrahlung Irradiation de contact Terapia proximal		60= 60= 60=	∿0.2 Cu ∿0.2 Cu ∿0.2 Cu	1.5 3 5	2-3 2-3 2-4.5	∿2000/8 mA ∿700/8 mA ∿300/8 mA	9 10 11
(van der Plaats)		50	∿0.2-3 Al	2-4	1-2.5	∿150-8000/2 mA	12

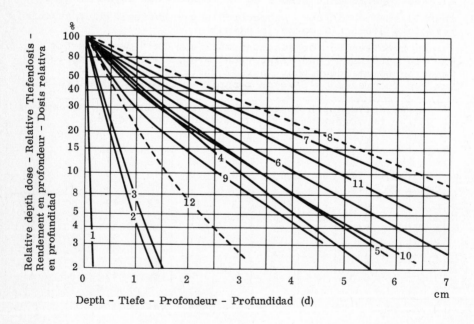

Depth - Tiefe - Profondeur - Profundidad (d)

Relative depth dose - Relative Tiefendosis -
Rendement en profondeur - Dosis relativa
en profundidad

4.2.8.4   Philips - Müller RT 100

Since many variations are possible, with this apparatus (as with
similar equipment), the following numbers must be regardet only
examples.

Da mit diesem Apparat - ebenso wie mit anderen ähnlichen - sehr vie-
le Variationen möglich sind, stellen folgende Zahlen nur Beispiele
dar.

Puisque de nombreuses variations sont possibles avec cet équipement
(ou avec des équipements semblables), les exemples suivants sont
donnés seulement à titre indicatif.

Puesto que con este aparato, lo mismo que con otros similares, son
posibles muchas variaciones, los siguientes ejemplos serán tomados
solamente como guía.

Method Methode Méthode Método	Tension Spannung Tension Tensión	Filter Filter Filtre Filtro	HVL HWSD CDA CHR	FSD FHA DFP DFP	Dose rate Dosisleistung Débit Intensidad	Curve Kurve Courbe Curva
(Therapy)	kV=	mm	mm Al	cm	R/min/mA	No
Grenz (Bucky) rays	10	∿1 Be	0.024	10	(100)	1
Grenzstrahlen	10	∿1 Be	0.024	30	12	1
	40	0.2 Al	0.15	15	110	2
Low energy	40	0.2 Al	0.15	30	28	3
Weichstrahl	50	0.5 Al	0.48	15	50	4
Rayons mous	50	0.5 Al	0.48	30	12	5
Rayos blandos	60	1.0 Al	1.0	15	32	6
Half deep	60	1.0 Al	1.0	30	8	7
Halbtief	100	0.5 Al	0.8	200	0.8	8
Semi profunde	100	0.2 Cu	0.2Cu	15	18	9
Semi profunda	100	0.2 Cu	0.2Cu	30	4.5	10

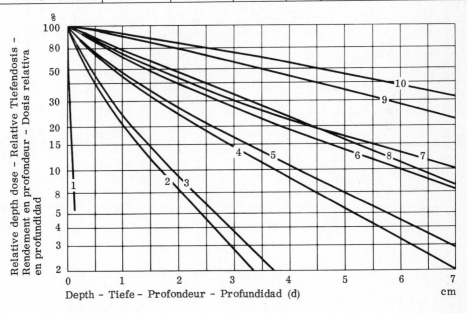

Relative depth dose - Relative Tiefendosis - Rendement en profondeur - Dosis relativa en profundidad

Depth - Tiefe - Profondeur - Profundidad (d)   cm

4.3   <u>Orthovoltage X-rays - Harte Röntgenstrahlen</u>
<u>Rayons X classiques - Rayos X duros</u>

4.3.1 <u>Relative depth doses - Relative Tiefendosen -</u>
<u>Rendements en profondeur - Dosis relativas en profundidad</u>

O.5 mm Cu HVL - HWSD - CDA - CHR

30 - 50 - 80 cm FSD - FHA - DFP - DFP

10-25-50-100-200-400 cm^2 Field size - Feld - Champ - Campo

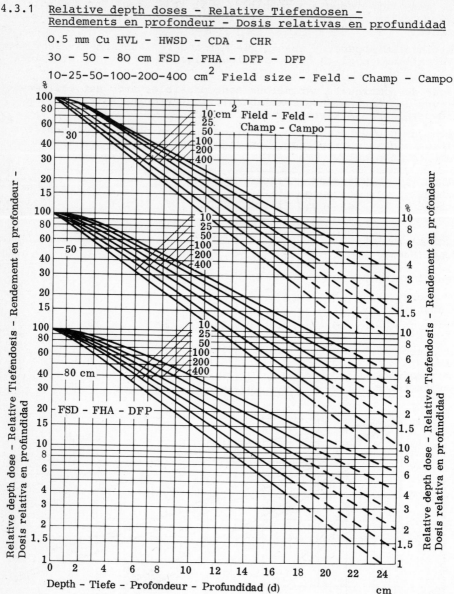

FSD FHA DFP	d cm	Field size - Feldgröße - Champ - Campo: 10	25	50	100	200	cm² 400
30 cm	0	100	100	100	100	100	100
	0.5	88	93	95	97	98	99
	1	80	85	91	94	96	97
	1.5	72	77	85	89	91	93
	2	65	70	78	84	86	89
	3	52	58	65	73	75	77
	4	43	48	54	61	64	66
	5	35	39	45	52	54	57
	6	28	32	38	43	46	49
	7	23	26	31	36	40	43
	8	18.5	22	26	31	34	37
	9	15.0	18.0	22	26	29	32
	10	12.5	15.0	18.0	21	25	28
	12	8.1	10.0	12.5	15.0	18.0	21
	14	5.4	6.8	8.8	11.0	13.5	14.0
	16	3.5	4.6	6.1	7.6	9.7	12.0
	18	2.4	3.1	4.3	5.3	7.2	8.9
	20	(1.5)	(2.1)	(3.0)	(3.7)	5.3	6.7
50 cm	0	100	100	100	100	100	100
	0.5	91	95	96	97	98	99
	1	83	88	92	95	97	98
	1.5	75	81	85	90	93	96
	2	68	76	80	85	90	93
	3	56	63	69	74	81	86
	4	46	53	59	65	72	77
	5	38	45	50	57	63	68
	6	32	38	43	48	55	59
	7	26	31	36	41	48	51
	8	22	26	30	35	41	45
	9	18.0	21	26	30	35	40
	10	15.0	18.0	22	26	31	35
	12	10.0	12.5	15.5	19.0	23	26
	14	6.6	8.4	11.5	13.5	17.0	20
	16	4.4	5.8	7.6	9.9	13.0	15.0
	18	3.0	4.0	5.5	7.1	9.3	11.5
	20	(2.0)	(2.8)	(3.9)	5.2	6.8	8.6
80 cm	0	100	100	100	100	100	100
	0.5	92	95	97	98	99	100
	1	86	89	92	95	97	99
	1.5	80	85	88	91	95	98
	2	73	79	83	87	91	94
	3	62	68	73	78	81	87
	4	52	58	63	69	73	79
	5	42	50	55	60	66	72
	6	35	42	46	52	58	66
	7	28	34	39	44	51	58
	8	24	29	33	38	45	51
	9	19.0	24	28	33	39	47
	10	16.0	20	24	28	34	41
	12	11.0	14.0	17.0	21	26	32
	14	7.4	9.8	12.5	15.0	19.5	25
	16	4.9	6.8	8.8	11.5	15.0	19.0
	18	(3.4)	(4.8)	(6.5)	(8.4)	11.5	15.0
	20	(2.2)	(3.3)	(4.6)	(6.1)	(8.7)	(12)

1 mm Cu HVL – HWSD – CDA – CHR

30 – 50 – 80 cm FSD – FHA – DFP – DFP

10-25-50-100-200-400 cm² Field size – Feld – Champ – Campo

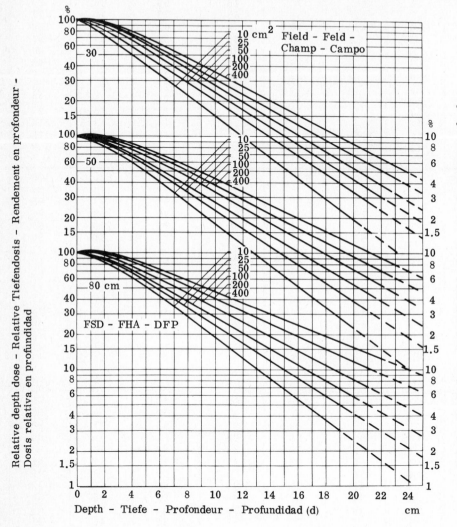

FSD FHA DFP	d cm	Field size - Feldgröße - Champ - Campo:					cm^2
		10	25	50	100	200	400
30 cm	0	100	100	100	100	100	100
	0.5	94	97	99	100	101	102
	1	89	93	97	99	101	102
	1.5	80	88	94	97	99	100
	2	73	82	88	93	94	97
	3	60	70	77	83	86	88
	4	50	58	66	73	76	80
	5	41	49	56	62	66	71
	6	34	42	47	53	57	62
	7	27	35	40	45	49	55
	8	22	29	34	38	42	48
	9	18.5	24	28	33	36	41
	10	15.0	20	24	28	31	36
	12	10.0	14.0	17.0	20	23	27
	14	6.6	9.8	12.5	14.5	17.0	20
	16	4.3	6.8	8.6	10.5	13.0	15.0
	18	2.9	4.8	6.1	7.6	9.5	11
	20	1.9	3.3	4.3	5.4	6.0	8.7
50 cm	0	100	100	100	100	100	100
	0.5	96	98	99	100	101	104
	1	91	95	97	99	101	104
	1.5	86	91	93	96	100	102
	2	81	86	89	94	97	100
	3	70	76	80	85	90	94
	4	60	67	70	77	82	86
	5	49	56	62	67	74	78
	6	40	47	52	60	66	70
	7	33	40	44	52	58	63
	8	27	33	37	45	50	56
	9	22	27	32	38	44	50
	10	17.5	23	27	33	38	44
	12	12.0	16.0	20	24	29	34
	14	7.8	11.5	14.0	18.0	22	26
	16	5.1	7.5	10.0	13.0	16.0	20
	18	3.4	5.3	7.4	9.8	12.5	15.0
	20	2.3	3.8	5.4	7.2	9.4	12.0
80 cm	0	100	100	100	100	100	100
	0.5	97	99	100	101	103	104
	1	94	97	99	101	104	105
	1.5	88	91	94	99	100	103
	2	84	88	90	95	98	101
	3	72	78	81	87	92	96
	4	61	67	71	77	85	88
	5	51	58	61	67	76	81
	6	42	48	52	59	67	72
	7	35	40	45	52	59	66
	8	28	34	38	45	52	58
	9	23	28	33	39	46	52
	10	19.0	24	28	34	41	47
	12	12.5	17.0	21	26	32	38
	14	8.4	12.0	15.0	19.5	25	30
	16	5.6	8.5	11.0	14.5	19.0	24
	18	3.4	6.0	8.0	11.0	15.0	19.5
	20	2.4	4.2	5.8	8.2	12.0	15.5

30 – 50 – 80 cm FSD – FHA – DFP – DFP

10-25-50-100-200-400 cm^2 Field size – Feld – Champ – Campo

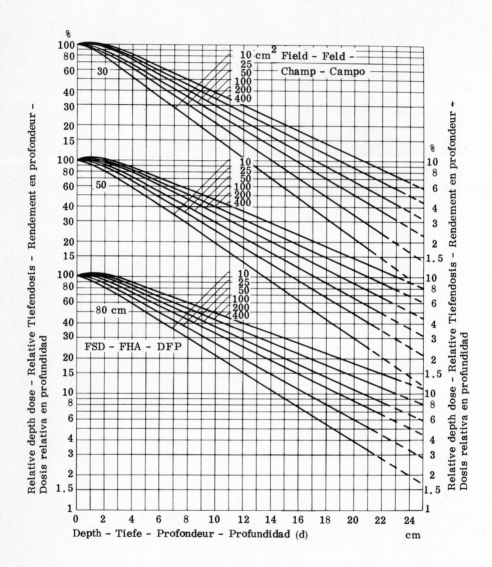

FSD FHA DFP	d cm	Field size – Feldgröße – Champ – Campo:					cm²
		10	25	50	100	200	400
30 cm	0	100	100	100	100	100	100
	0.5	95	96	97	100	102	104
	1	90	93	96	99	101	103
	1.5	83	88	92	97	99	102
	2	76	82	87	94	96	100
	3	63	72	76	84	88	92
	4	52	62	66	74	78	82
	5	43	51	57	63	67	72
	6	35	43	48	54	59	64
	7	28	36	41	46	52	56
	8	23	30	36	40	45	50
	9	19.5	25	30	34	39	44
	10	15.5	21	26	29	34	38
	12	10.5	14.5	19.0	22	26	30
	14	7.0	10.0	13.5	16.0	20	23
	16	4.7	7.0	9.7	12.5	15	18.0
	18	3.2	4.9	7.2	9.0	12	14.0
	20	2.2	3.4	5.1	6.6	8.8	11.0
50 cm	0	100	100	100	100	100	100
	0.5	95	98	100	102	104	105
	1	90	94	96	100	103	106
	1.5	85	92	95	98	101	105
	2	79	86	90	94	98	101
	3	68	76	80	87	92	96
	4	58	66	71	78	83	88
	5	49	56	62	68	74	79
	6	40	47	53	60	66	71
	7	33	40	46	53	58	64
	8	28	34	39	46	51	57
	9	23	29	34	40	45	51
	10	19.0	25	29	35	40	46
	12	13.0	18.0	22	26	31	37
	14	9.2	13.0	16.0	20	24	29
	16	6.3	9.3	12.0	15.0	19.0	33
	18	4.3	6.8	9.0	11.5	14.5	18.0
	20	3.0	4.9	6.6	7.7	11.5	14.5
80 cm	0	100	100	100	100	100	100
	0.5	96	98	100	102	104	106
	1	91	94	96	101	104	107
	1.5	86	92	98	100	104	107
	2	80	87	92	96	102	105
	3	69	75	83	89	94	99
	4	58	65	73	79	84	90
	5	49	57	64	70	75	80
	6	42	49	56	62	67	83
	7	35	42	49	54	60	66
	8	30	36	43	48	54	60
	9	25	31	38	42	48	54
	10	21	27	33	38	43	49
	12	15.0	20	25	29	34	40
	14	11.0	15.0	19.5	23	28	33
	16	7.8	11.0	15.0	18.0	22	27
	18	5.6	8.2	11.5	14.0	18.0	22
	20	3.9	6.0	8.8	11.0	14.0	18.0

<u>4 mm Cu HVL – HWSD – CDA – CHR</u>
30 – 50 – 80 cm FSD – FHA – DFP – DFP
10-25-50-100-200-400 cm^2 Field size – Feld – Champ – Campo

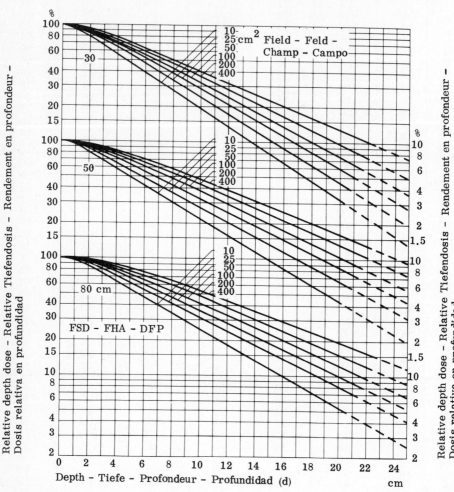

FSD FHA DFP	d cm	Field size - Feldgröße - Champ - Campo:					cm²
		10	25	50	100	200	400
30 cm	0	100	100	100	100	100	100
	0.5	95	96	97	98	99	100
	1	90	92	93	94	96	98
	1.5	85	88	90	92	94	96
	2	79	83	86	88	90	93
	3	66	74	77	79	83	87
	4	56	64	68	71	75	79
	5	47	54	60	63	66	71
	6	39	47	52	56	59	63
	7	33	40	44	48	51	57
	8	27	34	38	43	47	51
	9	23	28	33	37	41	45
	10	19.0	24	28	32	36	40
	12	13.5	17.0	21	24	28	32
	14	9.4	12.5	15.5	18.0	22	25
	16	6.6	8.4	11.5	13.5	16.5	20
	18	4.6	6.4	8.1	10.0	13.0	16.5
	20	(3.2)	4.5	5.9	6.6	9.6	13.0
50 cm	0	100	100	100	100	100	100
	0.5	98	98	99	99	100	100
	1	94	95	96	97	98	99
	1.5	86	90	92	94	96	98
	2	80	86	89	92	94	96
	3	68	75	80	84	87	90
	4	57	64	72	76	80	84
	5	49	56	63	68	73	77
	6	41	48	55	60	66	70
	7	35	42	48	54	59	65
	8	30	36	42	48	53	59
	9	25	31	37	43	48	53
	10	22	27	32	38	43	48
	12	16.0	20	25	29	34	38
	14	11.5	15.0	19.0	23	27	31
	16	8.1	11.5	14.5	17.5	21	25
	18	6.0	8.6	11.0	13.5	17.0	21
	20	(4.3)	6.3	8.4	10.5	13.0	16.0
80 cm	0	100	100	100	100	100	100
	0.5	98	98	99	99	100	101
	1	95	96	97	98	99	100
	1.5	91	94	96	97	99	100
	2	84	90	93	95	97	98
	3	74	80	85	88	91	93
	4	63	70	77	80	86	88
	5	54	62	68	73	78	83
	6	46	54	60	66	72	77
	7	40	47	53	59	65	70
	8	34	41	46	52	60	65
	9	29	36	41	46	53	58
	10	25	31	36	41	47	52
	12	18.0	24	28	33	38	44
	14	13.5	18.0	21	26	30	36
	16	9.8	13.5	16.5	20	24	29
	18	7.2	11.0	13.0	15.5	19.0	24
	20	5.2	8.0	9.8	12.5	15.0	19.0

4.3.5　Tissue-air ratio for orthovoltage X-rays
       Gewebe/Luft-Verhältnis für harte Röntgen-Strahlung
       Rapports tissu - air pour rayons X classiques
       Relación tejido/aire para rayos-X duros

1 mm Cu HVL - HWSD - CDA - CHR

0 - 400 cm^2 Field size - Feldgröße - Champ - Campo

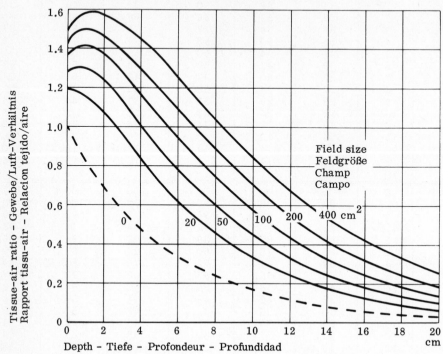

Depth - Tiefe - Profondeur - Profundidad

Depth Tiefe Profondeur Profundidad cm	Tissue-air ratio - Gewebe/Luft-Verhältnis - Rapport tissu - air - Relación tejido/aire					
	Field size - Feldgröße - Champ - Campo					cm^2
	0	20	50	100	200	400
0	1.0	1.19	1.23	1.33	1.41	1.50
1	0.81	1.16	1.30	1.42	1.50	1.59
2	0.69	1.08	1.24	1.37	1.46	1.57
3	0.58	0.96	1.14	1.27	1.38	1.53
4	0.48	0.83	1.00	1.16	1.28	1.46
5	0.39	0.72	0.89	1.05	1.19	1.36
6	0.33	0.63	0.79	0.95	1.09	1.25
7	0.28	0.54	0.70	0.85	0.98	1.14
8	0.24	0.46	0.60	0.75	0.88	1.04
9	0.20	0.39	0.53	0.66	0.78	0.94
10	0.17	0.34	0.45	0.58	0.70	0.85
12	0.12	0.24	0.33	0.44	0.55	0.68
14	0.08	0.18	0.24	0.33	0.41	0.54
16	0.06	0.12	0.18	0.25	0.33	0.43
18	0.04	0.09	0.14	0.18	0.25	0.33
20	0.03	0.06	0.10	0.13	0.18	0.26

2 mm Cu HVL - HWSD - CDA - CHR

O - 400 cm^2 Field size - Feldgröße - Champ - Campo

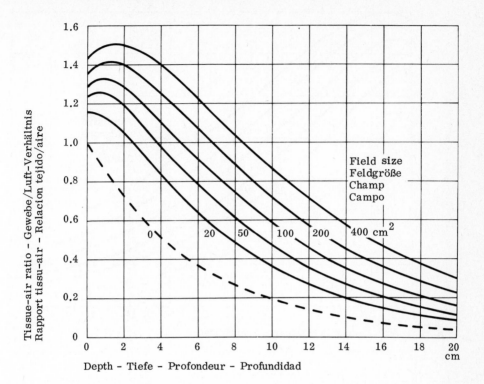

Depth - Tiefe - Profondeur - Profundidad

Depth Tiefe Profondeur Profundidad cm	Tissue-air ratio - Gewebe/Luft-Verhältnis - Rapport tissu-air - Relación tejido/aire					
	Field size - Feldgröße - Champ - Campo					cm^2
	O	20	50	100	200	400
O	1.0	1.16	1.23	1.29	1.35	1.42
1	0.85	1.13	1.25	1.33	1.42	1.49
2	0.73	1.05	1.19	1.29	1.39	1.49
3	0.61	0.94	1.08	1.20	1.33	1.47
4	0.51	0.83	0.98	1.10	1.24	1.40
5	0.43	0.73	0.88	1.00	1.16	1.32
6	0.37	0.64	0.79	0.91	1.07	1.22
7	0.31	0.56	0.70	0.83	0.98	1.12
8	0.27	0.49	0.62	0.75	0.88	1.04
9	0.23	0.42	0.54	0.66	0.80	0.95
10	0.19	0.36	0.47	0.59	0.72	0.87
12	0.14	0.27	0.36	0.46	0.57	0.71
14	0.10	0.20	0.27	0.35	0.45	0.58
16	0.07	0.15	0.21	0.27	0.36	0.46
18	0.05	0.11	0.16	0.21	0.28	0.38
20	0.04	0.09	0.12	0.16	0.23	0.30

Lit.: 1. ICRU, Rep. 10 a, Clin. Dosimetry, NBS-Handbook 87, Washington 1963
See page - Siehe Seite - Voir page - Ver página 114

3 mm Cu HVL - HWSD - CDA - CHR

O - 400 cm^2 Field size - Feldgröße - Champ - Campo

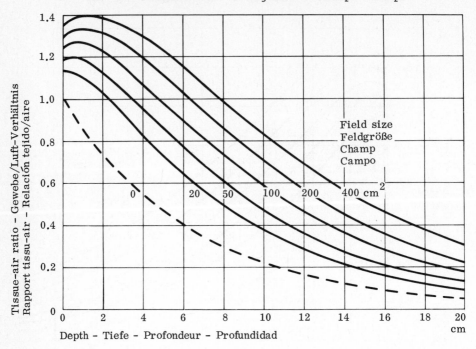

Depth - Tiefe - Profondeur - Profundidad

Depth Tiefe Profondeur Profundidad cm	Tissue-air ratio - Gewebe/Luft-Verhältnis - Rapport tissu-air - Relación tejido/aire					
	Field size - Feldgröße - Champ - Campo cm^2					
	O	20	50	1OO	2OO	4OO
O	1.OO	1.15	1.23	1.29	1.35	1.42
1	O.85	1.13	1.25	1.33	1.42	1.50
2	O.72	1.05	1.19	1.29	1.40	1.50
3	O.61	O.94	1.09	1.20	1.33	1.47
4	O.52	O.83	O.98	1.10	1.25	1.40
5	O.44	O.73	O.88	1.OO	1.15	1.32
6	O.37	O.64	O.79	O.92	1.07	1.22
7	O.31	O.56	O.70	O.82	O.98	1.12
8	O.26	O.49	O.62	O.74	O.88	1.04
9	O.23	O.43	O.54	O.66	O.79	O.95
1O	O.19	O.26	O.47	O.59	O.72	O.87
12	O.14	O.27	O.36	O.46	O.58	O.71
14	O.10	O.20	O.37	O.35	O.45	O.58
16	O.07	O.15	O.21	O.27	O.36	O.46
18	O.05	O.11	O.15	O.21	O.28	O.38
2O	O.04	O.09	O.12	O.16	O.23	O.30

Lit.: 2. SCHOKNECHT, G.: Strahlenther. 132, 516 (1967); 136, 24 (1968)
3. HOLT, J.G., LAUGHLIN, J.S., MORONEY, J.B.: Radiology 96, 437 (1970)

See page - Siehe Seite - Voir page - Ver pagina 115

4 mm Cu HVL - HWSD - CDA - CHR

O - 400 m^2 Field size - Feldgröße - Champ - Campo

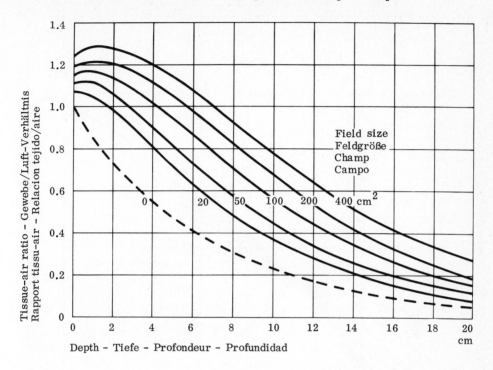

Depth - Tiefe - Profondeur - Profundidad

Depth Tiefe Profondeur Profundidad cm	Tissue-air ratio - Gewebe/Luft-Verhältnis - Rapport tissu-air - Relación tejido/aire					
	Field size - Feldgröße - Champ - Campo					cm^2
	O	20	50	100	200	400
O	1.00	1.07	1.11	1.15	1.19	1.24
1	0.85	1.05	1.12	1.17	1.22	1.29
2	0.73	0.98	1.06	1.14	1.20	1.27
3	0.63	0.90	0.98	1.08	1.16	1.24
4	0.54	0.81	0.90	1.02	1.12	1.20
5	0.47	0.72	0.81	0.95	1.05	1.14
6	0.41	0.63	0.73	0.87	0.97	1.07
7	0.36	0.55	0.65	0.78	0.90	1.00
8	0.31	0.48	0.57	0.70	0.83	0.93
9	0.27	0.42	0.51	0.63	0.75	0.85
10	0.23	0.37	0.45	0.56	0.68	0.98
12	0.17	0.28	0.34	0.45	0.53	0.64
14	0.13	0.21	0.26	0.35	0.42	0.52
16	0.09	0.16	0.20	0.26	0.33	0.41
18	0.07	0.11	0.15	0.20	0.25	0.34
20	0.05	0.07	0.12	0.16	0.18	0.27

Lit.: 4. COHEN, M., JONES, D.E.A., GREENE, D.: Central Axis Depth Dose Data for Use in Radiotherapy, Brit.J.Radiol., Suppl. 11 (1972)

4.4 Conversion of relative depth dose from 50 cm to other FSD's
Umrechnung relativer Tiefendosen von 50 cm auf andere FHA
Conversion de rendements en profondeur de 50 cm à d'autres DFP
Conversión de las dosis relativas en profundidad para 50 cm a
otras DFP

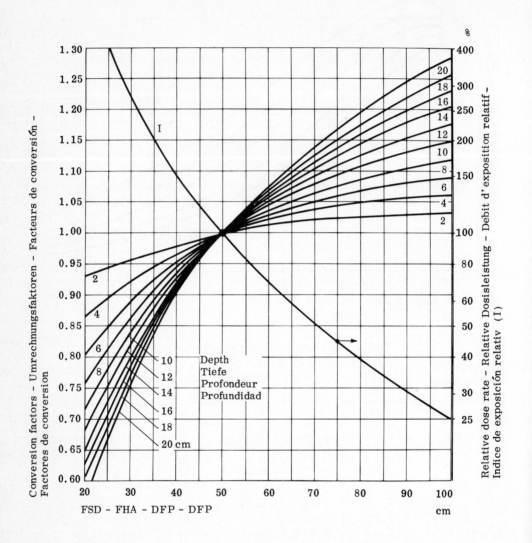

FSD - FHA - DFP - DFP

Lit.: 1. PFALZNER, P.M.: Brit.J.Radiol. 34, 236 (1961)
2. WEBSTER, E.W., TSIEN, K.C.: Atlas of Radiation Dose Distributions, IAEA, Vienna 1965
3. JOHNS, H.E., CUNNINGHAM, J.R.: The Physics of Radiology,
3th Edition, Springfield: Thomas 1969
4. BURNS, J.E., in: Depth Dose Data for Use in Radiotherapy,
Brit.J.Radiol., Suppl. 11, Appendix B, London 1972

FSD FHA DFP DFP cm	Conversion factors for tissue depths of Umrechnungsfaktoren für Gewebetiefen von Facteurs de conversion pour des profondeurs de Factores de conversión para profundidades en el tejido cm									
	2	4	6	8	10	12	14	16	18	20
20	0.93	0.86	0.81	0.76	0.72	0.68	0.65	0.63	0.60	–
25	0.95	0.90	0.85	0.82	0.78	0.75	0.73	0.71	0.69	0.66
30	0.96	0.92	0.89	0.86	0.80	0.82	0.80	0.79	0.77	0.76
35	0.97	0.95	0.93	0.91	0.89	0.88	0.86	0.86	0.85	0.84
40	0.98	0.96	0.95	0.95	0.94	0.93	0.92	0.92	0.91	0.91
45	0.99	0.98	0.98	0.97	0.97	0.97	0.97	0.96	0.96	0.96
50	1.00	1.00	1.00	1.00	1.00	1.00	1.00	1.00	1.00	1.00
55	1.01	1.01	1.01	1.02	1.02	1.03	1.03	1.03	1.04	1.04
60	1.01	1.02	1.03	1.04	1.04	1.05	1.06	1.06	1.07	1.08
65	1.02	1.03	1.04	1.05	1.06	1.07	1.08	1.09	1.10	1.11
70	1.02	1.04	1.05	1.06	1.08	1.09	1.11	1.12	1.13	1.14
75	1.03	1.05	1.06	1.08	1.10	1.11	1.13	1.14	1.15	1.17
80	1.03	1.05	1.07	1.09	1.11	1.13	1.14	1.16	1.18	1.20
85	1.03	1.06	1.08	1.10	1.12	1.14	1.16	1.18	1.20	1.22
90	1.03	1.06	1.08	1.11	1.13	1.16	1.18	1.20	1.25	1.25
95	1.03	1.06	1.09	1.11	1.14	1.17	1.20	1.22	1.24	1.27
100	1.03	1.06	1.09	1.12	1.15	1.18	1.21	1.23	1.26	1.29

Dose rate-Dosisleistung-Débit d'exposition-Indice de exposición: I

FSD - FHA - DFP cm (50 cm = 100 %)								
cm	20	25	30	35	40	45	55	60
I %	625	400	278	204	156	123	82.6	69.4
cm	65	70	75	80	85	90	95	100
I %	59.1	51.0	44.4	39.1	34.6	30.9	27.4	25

The conversion factors shown represent values which may be encounter-
ed in practice at different depths in tissue, when secondary effects
(scattering, finite focal spot size, etc.) are taken into account.
The conversion factors calculated from the inverse square law differ
to a small extend from those given above.

Die angegebenen Umrechnungsfaktoren stellen die in der Praxis unter
Berücksichtigung von sekundären Einflüssen (Streuung, endliche Fokus-
größe usw.) in verschiedenen Gewebetiefen etwa auftretenden Werte
dar. Die aus dem Quadratgesetz errechneten Umrechnungsfaktoren weichen von den angegebenen geringfügig ab.

Les facteurs de conversion donnés, représentent des valeurs rencon-
trées en pratique lorsque l'on tient compte des phénomènes secondaires (diffusion, dimensions du foyer, etc.). Les facteurs de conversion calculés par l'inverse carré des distances diffèrent un peu des
facteurs donnés ici.

Los factores de conversión indicados representan los valores practi-
cos teniendo en cuenta factores secundarios (dispersión, tamaño focal, etc.) en diferentes profundidades de tejido. Los valores teóri-
cos calculados a partir de la ley del cuadrado recíproco se apartan
de los aquí indicados dentro de ciertos límites.

4.5 γ-Teletherapy units - γ-Fernbestrahlungsapparaturen -
Appareils de télégammathérapie - Aparatos de telecurieterapia

4.5.1 <u>Cs 137</u>

15 - 20 - 30 - 40 - 50 cm SSD - QHA - DSP - DFP

100 cm^2 Field size - Feld - Champ - Campo

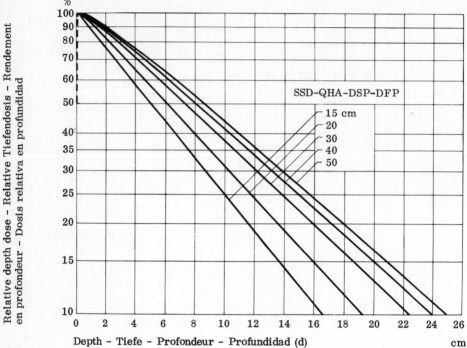

Depth - Tiefe - Profondeur - Profundidad (d)   cm

d cm	SSD - QHA - DSP - DFP					d cm	15	20	30	40	50
	15	20	30	40	50						
0	(50)	(50)	(50)	(50)	(50)	13	16.0	21	27	31	33
0.2	100	100	100	100	100	14	14.0	19.0	25	28	30
1	88	93	95	97	98	15	12.0	16.5	22	25	27
2	76	82	88	89	91	16	11.0	15.0	20	23	25
3	66	73	79	81	83	17	9.2	13.0	17.5	20	24
4	58	63	71	74	76	18	-	11.5	16.0	18.0	20
5	50	58	64	68	70	19	-	10.0	14.0	16.5	18.0
6	44	50	58	62	64	20	-	9.0	13.0	15.0	16.0
7	38	45	52	56	59	21	-	-	10.5	12.0	13.5
8	33	40	47	50	53	22	-	-	10.5	12.0	13.5
9	24	36	43	46	48	23	-	-	9.2	10.5	12.0
10	25	31	39	41	44	24	-	-	-	10.0	11.0
11	22	28	34	37	40	25	-	-	-	9.0	10.0
12	19	25	30	33	37						

Lit.: See page - Siehe Seite - Voir page - Ver página 119

4.5.2 Co 60

50 cm SSD - QHA - DSP - DFP

(O)-20-50-100-200-400 cm^2 Field size - Feld - Champ - Campo

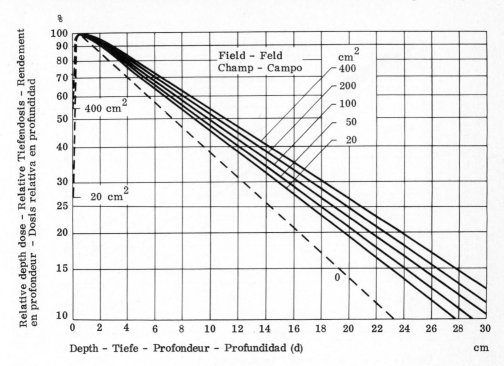

Depth - Tiefe - Profondeur - Profundidad (d)   cm

| Field size - Feldgröße - Champ - Campo: cm^2 | | | | | | | | | | | |
d cm	O	20	50	100	200	400	d cm	O	20	50	100	200	400
O	–	(29)	(36)	(43)	(58)	(55)	11	(34)	42	44	46	49	50
0.5	100	100	100	100	100	100	12	(31)	38	40	42	45	48
1	95	97	97	98	98	99	13	(28)	34	36	39	41	43
2	86	90	91	93	94	95	14	(26)	32	34	36	38	40
3	77	83	84	86	88	90	15	(23)	30	31	33	36	38
4	70	75	77	79	81	83	16	(21)	27	29	31	33	35
5	63	70	71	73	76	78	17	(19)	25	26	28	30	32
6	57	64	65	67	70	72	18	(17)	22	25	26	28	30
7	52	59	60	62	65	67	19	(15)	21	23	25	27	28
8	47	54	55	57	60	62	20	(14)	19.5	21	23	24	26
9	43	50	51	53	56	59	22	(12)	17.5	18.0	19.0	21	23
10	38	45	47	49	52	54	24	(9)	13.5	15.0	17.0	18.0	20

Lit.: 1. WEBSTER, E.W., TSIEN, K.C.: IAEA Atlas I, Vienna 1965
      2. DREXLER, G., WACHSMANN, F.: Strahlenther.132,1-7 (1967)
      3. COHEN, M., JONES, D.E.A., GREENE, D.: Central Axis Depth
         Dose Data for Use in Radiotherapy, Brit.J.Radiol.,
         Suppl. 11 (1972)

60 cm SSD – QHA – DSP – DFP

(O)-20-50-100-200-400 cm^2 Field size – Feld – Champ – Campo

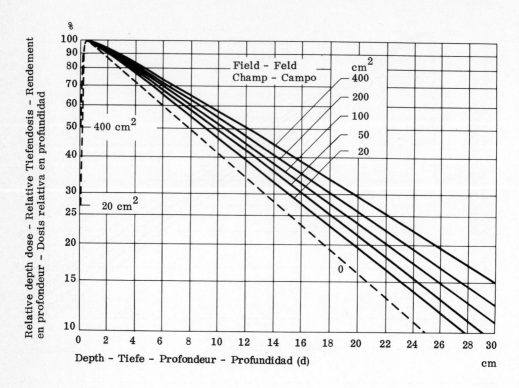

Relative depth dose – Relative Tiefendosis – Rendement en profondeur – Dosis relativa en profundidad

Depth – Tiefe – Profondeur – Profundidad (d)   cm

d cm	O	20	50	100	200	400	d cm	O	20	50	100	200	400
O	–	(26)	(32)	(36)	(42)	(50)	11	(38)	42	45	47	50	54
0.5	(100)	100	100	100	100	100	12	(34)	39	42	45	48	51
1	(94)	95	96	97	98	99	13	(31)	35	38	41	44	47
2	(87)	90	91	92	93	94	14	(28)	33	35	38	41	44
3	(79)	82	83	85	87	89	15	(25)	30	33	36	39	42
4	(71)	77	79	80	82	84	16	(23)	28	30	33	36	39
5	(64)	71	74	76	78	80	17	(20)	21	28	29	33	37
6	(60)	65	68	70	71	73	18	(19)	23	25	27	30	35
7	(53)	60	63	65	67	70	19	(18)	21	23	25	28	31
8	(49)	54	57	59	62	65	20	(16)	20	22	24	26	30
9	(45)	50	53	55	58	61	22	(13)	16.5	18.0	20	22	26
10	(41)	46	50	53	55	58	24	(11)	13.5	16.5	17.5	19.5	23

Field size – Feldgröße – Champ – Campo: cm^2

Co 60

80 cm SSD - QHA - DSP - DFP

(0)-20-50-100-200-400 cm^2 Field size - Feld - Champ - Campo

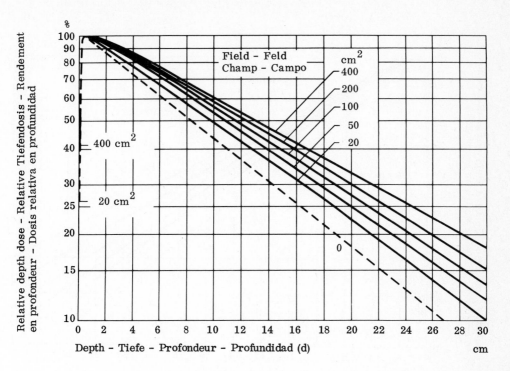

Relative depth dose - Relative Tiefendosis - Rendement en profondeur - Dosis relativa en profundidad

Depth - Tiefe - Profondeur - Profundidad (d)

cm

Field size - Feldgröße - Champ - Campo: cm^2											
d cm	0	20	50	100	200	400	d cm	0	20	50	100	200	400
0	–	(26)	(28)	(31)	(36)	(41)	11	40	45	50	53	55	57
0.5	100	100	100	100	100	100	12	37	43	45	49	52	54
1	95	97	97	98	98	99	13	33	40	43	45	47	50
2	87	90	92	94	96	97	14	31	37	40	42	45	47
3	80	84	88	90	91	92	15	28	34	37	40	43	45
4	73	78	82	84	86	87	16	26	32	34	37	40	43
5	67	72	77	79	81	83	17	24	28	32	34	37	40
6	62	67	72	74	76	77	18	22	27	29	32	35	37
7	57	63	67	70	72	73	19	20	25	28	30	33	36
8	52	58	63	65	67	68	20	18.0	23	25	28	30	34
9	47	54	58	61	63	64	22	15.0	19.0	22	24	27	29
10	43	50	53	56	59	61	24	13.0	16.0	18.5	21	23	26

<u>Co 60</u>

100 cm SSD - QHA - DSP - DFP

(0) -20-50-100-200-400 cm^2 Field size - Feld - Champ - Campo

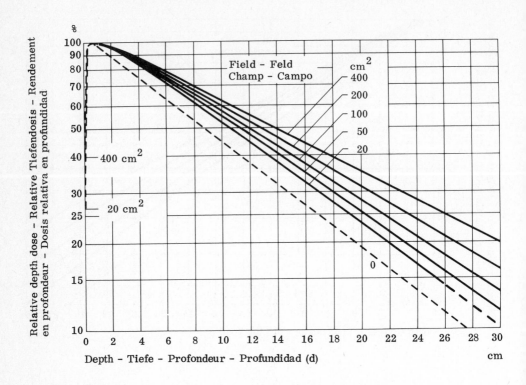

Depth - Tiefe - Profondeur - Profundidad (d)   cm

d cm	0	20	50	100	200	400	d cm	0	20	50	100	200	400
0	–	(25)	(28)	(31)	(36)	(40)	11	42	49	52	55	58	60
0.5	100	100	100	100	100	100	12	37	45	48	50	53	56
1	97	98	98	99	99	100	13	35	41	44	47	50	53
2	89	95	96	97	98	98	14	32	38	42	44	47	50
3	82	90	91	92	92	93	15	29	35	38	40	43	47
4	75	83	85	86	87	88	16	27	32	35	37	40	44
5	69	77	79	81	83	84	17	25	30	32	35	38	42
6	63	71	73	75	77	78	18	23	28	30	32	35	40
7	58	67	70	72	74	74	19	21	25	27	30	33	37
8	53	62	64	66	68	70	20	19.0	24	25	27	31	35
9	49	57	60	62	65	67	22	16.0	20	22	24	27	32
10	45	53	55	57	60	63	24	13.5	17.0	18.5	21	24	28

Field size - Feldgröße - Champ - Campo: cm^2

4.5.3   Tissue-air ratio for γ teletherapy units
         Gewebe/Luft-Verhältnis für γ-Fernbestrahlungsapparaturen
         Rapport tissu - air pour des appareils de télégamma-thérapie
         Relación tejido/aire para aparatos tele-γ

4.5.3.1 Cs 137

0 - 400 cm^2 Field size - Feldgröße - Champ - Campo

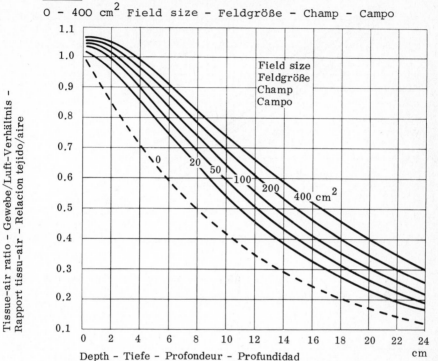

Depth - Tiefe - Profondeur - Profundidad

Depth Tiefe Profondeur Profundidad cm	Tissue-air ratio - Gewebe/Luft-Verhältnis - Rapport tissu-air - Relación tejido/aire					
	Field size - Feldgröße - Champ - Campo					cm^2
	0	20	50	100	200	400
0.2	1.00	1.02	1.04	1.05	1.06	1.07
1	0.93	1.00	1.02	1.04	1.05	1.06
2	0.85	0.96	0.99	1.02	1.04	1.05
3	0.78	0.91	0.95	0.98	1.00	1.03
4	0.72	0.86	0.90	0.93	0.97	0.99
5	0.65	0.80	0.85	0.89	0.92	0.95
6	0.59	0.75	0.79	0.84	0.88	0.91
7	0.55	0.70	0.74	0.79	0.83	0.87
8	0.50	0.64	0.69	0.74	0.78	0.83
9	0.46	0.59	0.64	0.69	0.74	0.78
10	0.42	0.54	0.59	0.65	0.69	0.74
12	0.35	0.46	0.51	0.56	0.61	0.66
14	0.29	0.39	0.44	0.48	0.54	0.59
16	0.25	0.33	0.37	0.41	0.47	0.52
18	0.21	0.27	0.32	0.36	0.41	0.46
20	0.17	0.23	0.27	0.30	0.35	0.40
22	0.14	0.19	0.23	0.26	0.30	0.35
24	0.12	0.16	0.18	0.22	0.26	0.30

4.5.3.2   Co 60

0 - 400 cm^2 Field size - Feldgröße - Champ - Campo

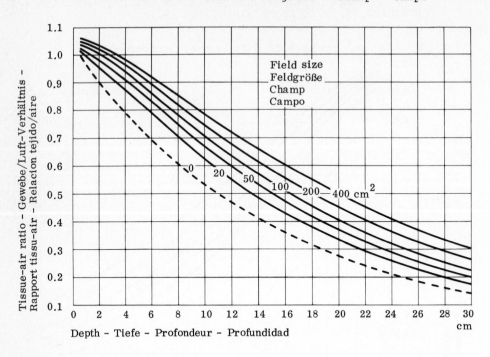

Depth - Tiefe - Profondeur - Profundidad

Depth Tiefe Profondeur Profundidad cm	Tissue-air ratio - Gewebe/Luft-Verhältnis - Rapport tissu-air - Relación tejido/aire					
	Field size - Feldgröße - Champ - Campo					cm^2
	0	20	50	100	200	400
0.5	1.00	1.02	1.03	1.04	1.05	1.06
2	0.91	0.96	0.98	1.00	1.02	1.03
4	0.79	0.86	0.91	0.94	0.96	0.98
6	0.69	0.79	0.83	0.86	0.89	0.92
8	0.61	0.71	0.75	0.78	0.82	0.85
10	0.54	0.62	0.67	0.71	0.75	0.78
12	0.47	0.55	0.60	0.64	0.68	0.72
14	0.42	0.48	0.53	0.57	0.62	0.66
16	0.36	0.43	0.48	0.51	0.56	0.60
18	0.32	0.38	0.42	0.46	0.50	0.55
20	0.28	0.34	0.38	0.41	0.45	0.60
22	0.24	0.30	0.33	0.37	0.41	0.46
24	0.21	0.26	0.29	0.33	0.37	0.41
26	0.18	0.23	0.26	0.29	0.33	0.37
28	0.16	0.20	0.23	0.26	0.29	0.34
30	0.14	0.18	0.20	0.22	0.26	0.31

Lit.: 1. COHEN, M., JONES, D.E.A., GREENE, D.: Central Axis Depth Dose Data for Use in Radiotherapy, Brit.J.Radiol., Suppl. 11 (1972)

4.6 Dose distributions obtainable with rotational irradiation
Mit Rotationsbestrahlung erreichbare Dosisverteilungen
Distributions de doses obtenues en cyclothérapie
Distribución de la dosis asequible mediante radiación rotatoria

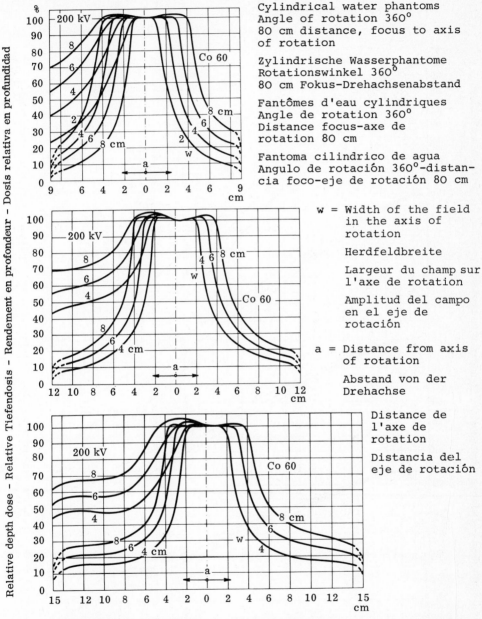

Cylindrical water phantoms
Angle of rotation 360°
80 cm distance, focus to axis
of rotation

Zylindrische Wasserphantome
Rotationswinkel 360°
80 cm Fokus-Drehachsenabstand

Fantômes d'eau cylindriques
Angle de rotation 360°
Distance focus-axe de
rotation 80 cm

Fantoma cilíndrico de agua
Angulo de rotación 360°-distan-
cia foco-eje de rotación 80 cm

w = Width of the field
in the axis of
rotation

Herdfeldbreite

Largeur du champ sur
l'axe de rotation

Amplitud del campo
en el eje de
rotación

a = Distance from axis
of rotation

Abstand von der
Drehachse

Distance de
l'axe de
rotation

Distancia del
eje de rotación

Lit.: 1. WACHSMANN, F., BARTH, G.: Bewegungsbestrahlung, Stuttgart:
Thieme 1953
2. WACHSMANN, F., BARTH, G., LANZL, L.H., CARPENDER, W.J.:
Moving Field Therapy, University of Chicago Press 1962

Percentage depth doses with supervoltage X-rays
Relative Tiefendosen sehr harter Röntgenstrahlen
Rendements en profondeur, rayonnements de haute énergie
Dosis relativas en profundidad para radiaciones muy duras

1 - 2 - 5 - 10 MV

100 cm FSD - FHA - DFP - DFP

25 - 100 - 225 cm^2 Field size - Feld - Champ - Campo

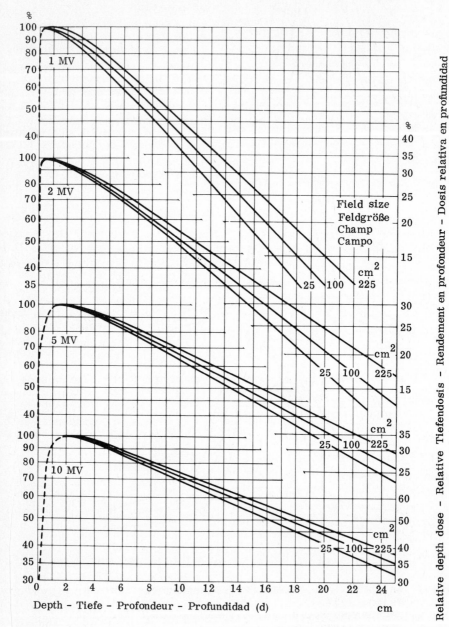

Relative depth dose – Relative Tiefendosis – Rendement en profondeur – Dosis relativa en profundidad

Depth - Tiefe - Profondeur - Profundidad (d)   cm

d cm	Field size - Feld - Champ - Campo 25	100	225	25	100	225 cm²
	Relative depth dose - Relative Tiefendosis - Rendement en profondeur - Dosis relativa en profundidad %					
	1 MV			2 MV		
0	(45)	(55)	(70)	(29)	(39)	(55)
0.5	99	100	100	99	100	100
1	97	98	99	98	99	99
2	90	93	97	94	94	95
3	81	85	90	88	89	91
4	73	78	83	81	83	85
5	65	71	76	74	76	79
6	59	64	70	69	71	73
7	52	57	62	63	65	68
8	47	52	57	57	60	62
9	41	45	49	52	55	58
10	36	40	45	48	50	53
11	32	36	41	43	46	49
12	27	32	37	39	42	46
13	24	28	33	36	39	42
14	21	25	29	32	36	39
15	18.0	22	26	28	32	37
16	15.5	19.0	23	26	29	34
17	13.5	17.0	21	23	27	31
18	12.0	15.0	18.5	21	24	29
(19)	10.5	13.0	17.0	19.0	22	26
20	9.0	12.0	15.0	17.0	20	24
22	-	9.0	12.0	14.0	17.0	21
24	-	-	9.0	12.5	14.5	19.5
	5 MV			10 MV		
0	(20)	(28)	(35)	(16)	(22)	(27)
0.5	(78)	(80)	(84)	(67)	(75)	(78)
1	(97)	(98)	(99)	(90)	(92)	(94)
1.5	100	100	100	(96)	(97)	(98)
2	98	99	99	99	99	99
2.5	97	98	99	100	100	100
3	95	97	98	98	99	99
4	90	92	94	93	95	97
5	86	88	91	89	91	93
6	81	83	86	85	87	89
7	76	78	81	80	82	84
8	72	74	77	77	79	81
9	67	70	73	72	75	77
10	63	66	69	69	71	73
11	58	62	64	65	68	71
12	54	57	61	62	65	68
13	51	54	57	58	62	64
14	48	51	54	55	59	62
15	45	48	52	53	56	59
16	42	45	48	51	53	56
17	39	42	46	48	51	54
18	37	40	43	46	49	52
19	35	38	41	43	46	49

Lit.: 1. WEBSTER, E.W., TSIEN, K.C.: IAEA Atlas of Radiation Dose
Distributions, Vol. I, Vienna 1965
2. COHEN, M., JONES, D.E.A., GREENE, D.: Brit.J.Radiol.,
Suppl. 11 (1972)

4.8.1   Percentage depth doses for very high energy X-rays
Relative Tiefendosen ultraharter Röntgenstrahlen
Rendements en profondeur, rayonnements X de très haute energie
Dosis relativas en profundidad para radiaciones X ultraduras

15 - 20 - 30 - 50 - 100 MV

50 - 75 - 100 cm FSD - FHA - DFP - DFP

(15-) 100 (-400) cm^2 Field size - Feldgröße - Champ - Campo

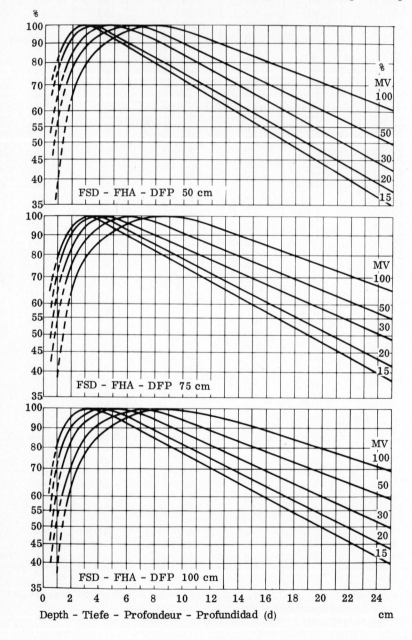

Relative depth dose - Relative Tiefendosis - Rendement en profondeur - Dosis relativa en profundidad   %

d cm	Quality - Qualität - Qualité - Calidad										MV
	15	20	30	50	100		15	20	30	50	100
0	(20)	(16)	(15)	(13)	(10)		(20)	(16)	(15)	(13)	(10)
0.5	(66)	(63)	(55)	(42)	(21)		(66)	(61)	(53)	(41)	(20)
1	(82)	(76)	(67)	(57)	40		78	(72)	(63)	(55)	(38)
1.5	90	85	75	(64)	(50)		88	82	74	(67)	(51)
2	97	93	85	77	65		94	90	82	75	64
2.5	99	97	90	83	72		97	95	90	81	72
3	100	98	94	88	78		100	98	94	87	78
3.5	98	100	98	92	84		99	99	97	91	87
4	97	99	99	94	88		98	100	99	94	86
4.5	94	97	100	97	91		96	98	100	96	89
5	92	94	100	98	92		93	97	99	98	92
6	88	90	98	100	97		90	92	97	100	97
7	84	86	95	99	99		85	89	92	98	98
8	80	82	92	97	100		82	86	90	97	100
9	76	78	88	93	99		78	82	87	94	100
10	72	75	84	90	97		75	78	84	91	99
11	68	72	80	87	95		72	75	80	88	98
12	65	68	76	83	92		68	72	78	85	95
13	62	65	73	80	88		65	68	85	87	92
14	59	62	70	77	86		63	66	72	80	90
15	56	59	67	74	83		60	63	70	77	88
16	53	57	64	70	80		57	61	67	74	85
17	51	54	61	68	78		55	58	65	72	82
18	48	52	58	65	75		52	56	63	69	80
19	46	49	56	63	73		50	53	61	67	78
20	44	47	53	60	72		48	52	58	75	85
21	42	45	51	58	68		46	49	57	63	74
22	40	43	48	56	67		43	47	54	61	71
23	38	41	46	58	65		42	45	52	59	68
24	37	39	44	52	63		40	43	51	57	67
25	35	37	42	50	60		38	42	48	55	65

(Left block: FSD - FHA - DFP 50 cm; Right block: FSD - FHA - DFP 75 cm)

d cm	Quality - Qualität -					d cm	Qualité - Calidad				MV
	15	20	30	50	100		15	20	30	50	100
0	(20)	(16)	(15)	(13)	(10)	11	74	78	94	92	98
0.5	(65)	(60)	(52)	(40)	(20)	12	71	75	82	89	96
1	81	(71)	(62)	(53)	(38)	13	68	73	78	86	95
1.5	90	80	71	60	(50)	14	65	69	75	83	93
2	95	90	82	70	62	15	62	66	72	81	91
2.5	98	93	88	76	69	16	60	64	69	78	89
3	99	97	92	84	76	17	57	62	67	76	87
3.5	100	98	95	88	81	18	54	58	65	73	84
4	98	100	97	92	85	19	52	56	62	71	82
4.5	97	99	99	94	88	20	50	54	60	79	80
5	96	98	100	96	91	21	47	52	58	67	77
6	92	95	99	98	95	22	46	50	55	65	75
7	89	92	97	100	98	23	44	48	53	63	73
8	85	89	95	99	100	24	42	46	52	61	71
9	81	85	91	97	100	25	40	43	49	59	69
10	78	82	88	94	99						

(Left block: FSD - FHA - DFP 100 cm)

See page - Siehe Seite - Voir page - Ver página 126

4.8.2 Angular distribution of megavoltage X-rays
Winkelverteilung ultraharter Röntgenstrahlen
Distribution angulaire des rayons X de très haute énergie
Reparto angular de radiaciones ultraduras

Average values - Richtwerte - Valeurs moyennes -
Valores aproximados

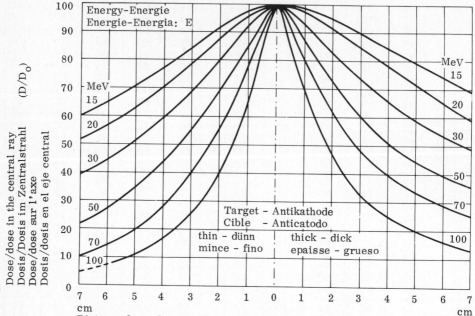

Distance from the central ray at 100 cm FD - Abstand vom Zentralstrahl in
100 cm FA - Distance à l'axe à DF 100 cm - Distancia del rayo central en
100 cm DF = d

| d | D/D₀ Target - Antikathode - Cible - Anticàtodo | | | | | | | | | | | %|
| | Thin - Dünn - Mince - Fino E MeV | | | | | | Thick-Dick-Épaisse-Grueso E MeV | | | | | |
cm	15	20	30	50	70	100	15	20	30	50	70	100
0	100	100	100	100	100	100	100	100	100	100	100	100
0.5	99	98	97	94	90	83	100	99	97	95	92	85
1	98	96	92	85	78	65	99	97	93	87	80	70
1.5	95	94	87	77	65	51	97	95	87	80	71	57
2	92	88	80	69	55	40	95	92	83	73	61	47
2.5	88	83	74	62	47	32	93	88	78	66	54	39
3	84	79	69	56	40	25	90	85	74	60	49	33
4	77	74	60	44	28	17	85	78	65	51	40	25
5	71	63	52	35	20	11	80	72	59	45	34	20
6	65	57	45	27	14	(7)	75	65	53	40	29	16
7	60	51	39	21	10	(5)	69	60	49	35	25	13

Lit.: 1. CHARLTON, E.K., BREED, H.E.: Am.J.Roentgenol. 60, 158 (1948)
2. GUND, K., SCHITTENHELM, R.: Strahlenther. 92, 506 (1953)

4.8.3 Approximate relative depth dose of X- and γ-rays at a depth
of O and 0.5 cm, and depth of the dose maximum (summary)

Ungefähre rel. Tiefendosen von Röntgen- und γ-Strahlen in O
und 0,5 cm und Tiefenlage des Dosismaximums (Zusammenfassung)

Dose approximative de rayons X et γ à une profondeur de O et
0,5 cm et profondeur de la dose maximale (résumé)

Dosis rel.en profundidad aproximada de rayos X y γ a profundidades de O y 0,5 cm y profundidad de la dosis máxima
(resumen)

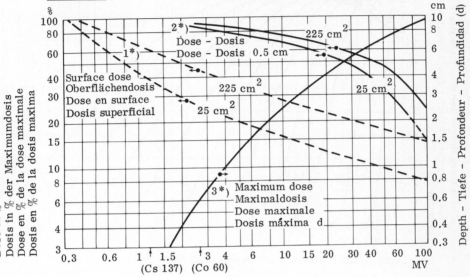

Energy - Energie - Energie - Energía

Energy Energie Energie Energía	1. Surface dose *) Oberfl. Dosis Dose en surface Dosis superficial		2. Dose at *) Dosis in Dose à Dosis en: 0.5 cm		3. Dose max. *) Max. Dosis Dose max. Dosis max.
MV	25 cm² %	225 cm²	25 cm² %	225 cm²	d cm
0.3	100	100	–	–	(∿0)
0.5	(70)	(92)	–	–	(∿0)
1.0	(44)	(65)	–	–	(0.1)
Cs 137	(39)	(61)	–	–	(0.17)
1.5	(34)	(55)	–	–	0.26
Co 60	(26)	(45)	87	90	0.60
5	(20)	(38)	77	84	1.35
10	(16)	(29)	68	77	2.5
20	(13)	(23)	58	67	4.1
30	(12)	(20)	47	58	5.5
50	(8)	(17)	32	47	7.0
100	(7)	(15)	24	(15)	9.5

Lit.: See pages - Siehe Seiten - Voir pages - Ver páginas 118-129
*) See graph - Siehe Abbildung - Voir image - Ver gráfica

4.9   Relative depth doses of high-energy-electrons
Relative Tiefendosen schneller Elektronen
Rendements en profondeur pour des électrons accélérés
Dosis relativas para electrones de alta energía

4.9.1   1 - 10 MeV Energy - Energie - Énergie - Energía

(40) - 60 - (80) cm SSD - QHA - DSP - DFP

(10) - 50 - (100) cm^2 Field - Feld - Champ - Campo

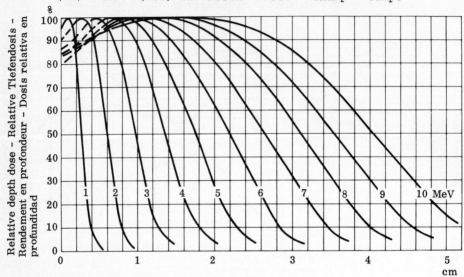

Depth - Tiefe - Profondeur - Profundidad (d)

d	Depth doses as % of the maximum dose - Tiefendosis in % der Maximaldosis -Rendement en profondeur en % de la dose maximum Dosis en profundidad en % de la dosis máxima									
	Energy - Energie - Énergie - Energía:									MeV
cm	1	2	3	4	5	6	7	8	9	10
0	(96)	(90)	(87)	(83)	(80)	(82)	(83)	(84)	(85)	(86)
0.1	100	(95)	(83)	(87)	(82)	(84)	(84)	(85)	(86)	(87)
0.2	83	(98)	(91)	(88)	(86)	(86)	(86)	(87)	(89)	(90)
0.3	34	100	(96)	(91)	(88)	(89)	(88)	(89)	(91)	(91)
0.4	8	94	(99)	(94)	(92)	(91)	(90)	(92)	(94)	(93)
0.6	(1)	50	97	(99)	(98)	(94)	(93)	(96)	(95)	(94)
0.8	−	10	80	98	100	(99)	(98)	(99)	(96)	(96)
1.0	−	(1)	47	89	98	100	100	100	(98)	(97)
1.2	−	−	17	69	94	98	100	100	(99)	(98)
1.4	−	−	4.5	4.5	82	92	98	100	100	(99)
1.6	−	−	(2)	22	66	84	94	98	100	100
1.8	−	−	−	10	46	74	88	96	99	100
2.0	−	−	−	4	26	62	81	92	96	99
2.5	−	−	−	(2)	4	30	58	76	87	93
3.0	−	−	−	−	(2)	4	32	55	72	80
3.5	−	−	−	−	−	(2)	9	31	51	68
4.0	−	−	−	−	−	−	(3)	10	30	48
5.0	−	−	−	−	−	−	−	−	(4)	12

4.9.2　10 - 100 MeV Energy - Energie - Energie - Energía

(40) - 60 - (100) cm　SSD - QHA - DSP - DFP

(15) - 100 - (200) cm^2 Field area - Feld - Champ - Campo

Relative depth dose - Relative Tiefendosis - Rendement en profondeur - Dosis relativa en profundidad

Depth - Tiefe - Profondeur - Profundidad (d)

d	Depth doses as % of the maximum dose - Tiefendosis in % der Maximaldosis - Rendement en profondeur en % de la dose maximum - Dosis en profundidad en % de la dosis máxima									
	Energy - Energie - Énergie - Energía									MeV
cm	10	15	20	25	30	40	50	60	70	100
0	(86)	(87)	(88)	(88)	(88)	(89)	(88)	(88)	(87)	(85)
1	(97)	(96)	(95)	(94)	(93)	(93)	(92)	(91)	(90)	(88)
2	99	100	100	(99)	(99)	(97)	(96)	(95)	(94)	(92)
3	80	97	99	100	100	(98)	(98)	(98)	(96)	(94)
4	48	88	97	99	100	(99)	(99)	(99)	(98)	(96)
5	12	70	90	96	97	100	100	100	99	(99)
6	2	50	79	88	94	98	99	100	100	(100)
7	–	28	63	78	88	95	99	98	99	(100)
8	–	7	44	68	81	91	96	97	97	(99)
9	–	3	26	55	72	85	93	94	96	(99)
10	–	–	9	40	61	78	88	92	94	(98)
12	–	–	3	12	39	64	77	83	87	(96)
14	–	–	–	4	17	50	66	74	81	(90)
16	–	–	–	6	5	34	54	64	73	(84)
18	–	–	–	–	–	18	42	53	63	(78)
20	–	–	–	–	–	7	29	42	53	(72)
22	–	–	–	–	–	–	18	31	42	(64)
24	–	–	–	–	–	–	10	21	32	(57)
26	–	–	–	–	–	–	8	13	22	(52)

Lit.: 1. GUND, K., WACHSMANN, F.: Strahlenther. 7, 573 (1948)
2. LAUGHLIN, J.S. et al.: Radiology 60, 165 (1953)
3. WEBSTER, E.W., TSIEN, K.C.: Atlas of Radiation Dose Distributions, IAEA, Vienna 1965
4. COHEN, M., JONES, D.E.A., GREENE, D.: Brit.J.Radiol., Suppl. 11 (1972)

4.10   <u>Relative depth doses for heavy particles</u>
        <u>Relative Tiefendosen schwerer Teilchen</u>
        <u>Rendements en profondeur pour des particules lourdes</u>
        <u>Dosis relativas en profundidad de particulas pesadas</u>

4.10.1 <u>Neutrons - Neutronen - Neutrons - Neutrones</u>

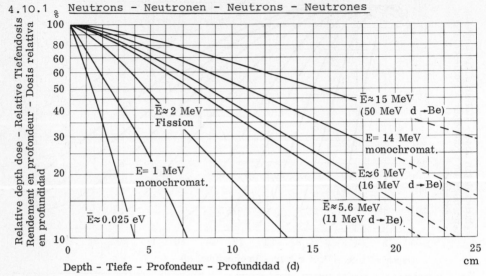

Depth - Tiefe - Profondeur - Profundidad (d)

d	Relative depth dose - Relative Tiefendosis - Rendement en profondeur - Dosis relativas en profundidad						
	Energy - Energie - Energie - Energía						
cm	$\bar{E}\approx$ 0.025 eV	E= 1 MeV	$\bar{E}\approx$ 2 MeV	$\bar{E}\approx$ 5.6 MeV	$\bar{E}\approx$ 6 MeV	E= 14 MeV	$\bar{E}\approx$ 15 MeV
0.5	76	87	97	98	98	99	100
1	60	76	91	94	96	98	99
1.5	45	66	86	92	94	96	98
2	30	57	80	88	90	94	97
3	19	43	68	81	83	88	93
4	10	32	57	73	77	83	89
5	–	24	47	66	71	78	85
6	–	16	40	60	65	73	82
7	–	11	33	53	59	67	78
8	–	–	27	48	53	63	74
10	–	–	18	38	43	53	66
12	–	–	13	30	35	46	60
14	–	–	–	24	28	39	54
16	–	–	–	19	23	33	48
18	–	–	–	15	18	28	43
20	–	–	–	(12)	(15)	(23)	(38)
22	–	–	–	–	(12)	(20)	(35)
24	–	–	–	–	–	(17)	(30)

Lit.: 1. BEWLEY, D.K.: Current Topics in Rad.Res., Amsterdam: North-
          Holland Publ.Co. (1970)
       2. SNYDER, W.S.: NCRP Report No. 38, Washington (1971)
       3. BROERSE, J.J. et al. in: Proc. First Symp. on Neutron Dosi-
          metry, München (1972) (EUR 4896 dfe)
       4. Brit.J.Radiol., Suppl. <u>11</u> (1972)

4.10.2 Protons, α-particles and mesons
        Protonen, α-Teilchen und Mesonen
        Protons, particules α et mésons
        Protones, particulas α y mesones

    1. 140 MeV Protons - Protonen - Protons - Protones
       1 - (12) cm Ø Field size - Feld - Champ - Campo 3)

    2. 570-605 MeV α-Particles-Teilchen-Particules-Particulas
       1- (2) cm Ø Field size - Feld - Champ - Campo 4)

    3. 84 MeV π- Mesons - Mesonen - Mésons - Mesones
       1- (2) cm Ø Field size - Feld - Champ - Campo 2)

    4. 58 - 77 MeV π- Mesons - Mesonen - Mésons - Mesones
       (1) - 5 cm Ø Field size - Feld - Champ - Campo 5)

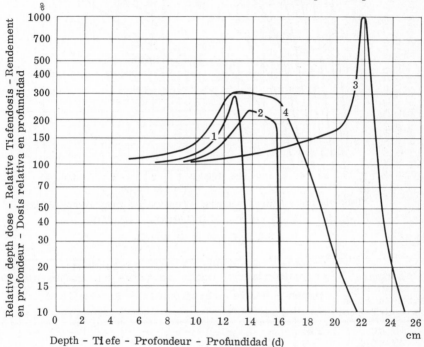

Depth - Tiefe - Profondeur - Profundidad (d)

Note - Bemerkung - Remarque - Nota:

The "biologic depth dose curves" have a different shape because the
RBE of these radiations changes considerably with depth.

Die "biologischen Tiefendosiskurven" haben der sich mit der Tiefe
stark ändernden RBW dieser Strahlungen wegen einen anderen Verlauf.

Les "courbes d'effet biologique en profondeur" ont une forme très
différente car l'EBR de ces particules varie beaucoup en profondeur.

Las "curvas de dosis profundas biológicas" son distintas porque la
EBR varia considerablemente con la profundidad.

Lit.: 1. CURTIS, S.C., RAJU, M.R.: Rad.Res. 34, 239 (1968)
      2. ALSMILLER, R.G. et al.: Nucl.Sci.Eng. 43, 257 (1971)
      3. KOEHLER, A.M., PRESTON, W.M.: Rad.Phys. 104, 191 (1972)
      4. ALSMILLER, R.G. et al.: ORNL-TM-4369 (1974)
      5. ARMSTRONG, T.W., CHANDLER, K.C.: Rad.Res. 58, 293 (1974)

4.11 Relative depth dose at different depths in tissue (water)
      Relative Tiefendosen in verschiedenen Gewebe-(Wasser-)Tiefen
      Rendements à différentes profondeurs de tissu (eau)
      Dosis relativas a diferentes profundidades de tejido (agua)

50 cm FSD - FHA - DFP - DFP

100 cm^2 Field size - Feldgröße - Champ - Campo

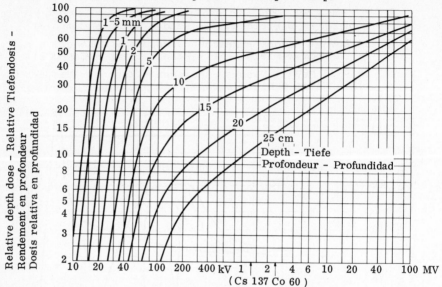

Tube voltage - Röhrenspannung - Tension d'alimentation - Voltaje del tubo

0.01 0.1   1   5   10 mm Al HVL-HWSD-CDA-CHR

0.3 1 2 4 6 8 10 mm Cu

Tube voltage Röhrenspannung Tension du tube Voltaje del tubo	Relative depth dose - Rel. Tiefendosis - Rendement en profondeur - Dosis relativa en profundidad %								
	Depth - Tiefe - Profondeur - Profundidad								
	1	5 mm	1	2	5	10	15	20	25 cm
10 kV	2.8	–	–	–	–	–	–	–	–
20 kV	70	44	10	–	–	–	–	–	–
30 kV	90	75	41	17	3.6	–	–	–	–
50 kV	99	91	76	53	23	7.5	2.8	–	–
100 kV	∿100	(98)	92	81	51	23	11	4.5	–
200 kV	∿100	∿100	(99)	95	68	33	17	8.4	4.3
300 kV	∿100	∿100	∿100	(98)	73	37	20	10	5.8
500 kV	∿100	∿100	∿100	(99)	76	42	24	13	7.6
1 MV	∿100	∿100	∿100	∿100	83	49	29	16	10
2 MV	∿100	∿100	∿100	∿100	87	52	35	22	12
4 MV	∿100	∿100	∿100	∿100	(92)	58	40	27	17
10 MV	∿100	∿100	∿100	∿100	∿100	67	48	36	25
20 MV	∿100	∿100	∿100	∿100	∿100	74	57	44	33
50 MV	∿100	∿100	∿100	∿100	∿100	83	70	59	48
100 MV	∿100	∿100	∿100	∿100	∿100	90	80	73	62

Lit.: See pages - Siehe Seiten - Voir pages - Ver paginas 87 - 99,
      104 - 111, 118 - 122, 126 - 129

Table of contents - Inhaltsverzeichnis
Table des matières - Tabla de materias

5.1   Back scatter of X- and gamma rays
           Rückstreuung von Röntgen- und Gammastrahlung
           Rétrodiffusion de rayons X et gamma
           Retrodispersión de rayos X y gamma

           10 kV - Co 60

           20 - 400 cm^2 Field size - Feld - Champ - Campo

5.1.1   Quadratic or circular fields - Quadratische oder kreisrunde
           Felder - Champs carrés ou circulaires - Campos cuadrados o
           circulares

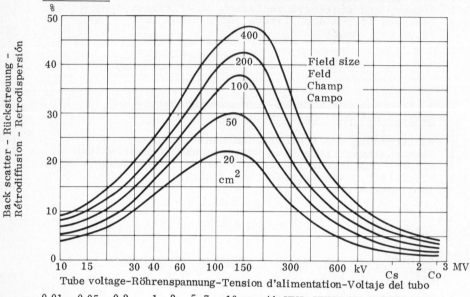

Radiation quality Strahlenqualität Qualité du rayonnement Calidad de la radiación		Back scatter - Rückstreuung - Rétrodiffusion - Retrodispersión % Field area - Feld - Champ - Campo cm^2				
kV-MV	HVL-HWSD-CDA-CHR	20	50	100	200	400
10 kV	0.013 mm Al	3.8	5.3	6.8	8.0	9.0
15 kV	0.045 " "	5.3	6.7	8.2	10.0	11.5
20 kV	0.10 " "	6.6	8.4	10.4	12.5	14.5
30 kV	0.35 " "	10.0	12.0	15.0	17.0	20
50 kV	1.7 " "	15.5	20	23	26	29
70 kV	4.0 " "	19.0	24	28	31	36
100 kV	8 mm Al 0.3 mm Cu	22	29	34	39	44
150 kV	0.8 mm Cu	22	29	37	42	48
200 kV	1.8 " "	18.0	25	32	40	46
300 kV	3.8 " "	11.5	16.0	20	26	34
400 kV	5.5 " "	8.0	11.5	15.0	18.0	24
600 kV	7.7 " "	5.0	7.0	9.5	12.5	15.5
1 MV	10 " "	2.2	4.0	5.8	7.4	9.3
Cs 137	–	1.7	2.9	4.4	5.9	7.2
2 MV	–	1.3	2.2	3.2	4.3	5.3
Co 60	–	1.2	1.8	2.6	3.5	4.3

5.1.2 Back scatter in the case of non-square fields
Rückstreuung bei nicht quadratischen Feldern
Rétrodiffusion par champs non-carrés
Retrodispersión con campos no cuadrados

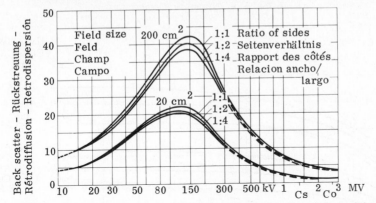

Tube voltage-Röhrenspannung-Tension d'alimentation-Voltaje del tubo

0.01 0.1   1 2 5 8 mm Al HVL-HWSD-CDA-CHR

0.3 1 2 3 5 6 8 10 mm Cu

Radiation quality Strahlenqualität Qualité du rayonnement Calidad de la radiación			Back scatter - Rückstreuung - Rétrodiffusion - Retrodispersión %					
Tube Röhre Ampoule Tubo	HVL - HWSD CDA - CHR		Field size and ratio of sides - Feldgröße und Seitenverhältnis - Dimensions du champ et rapport des côtés - Tamaño del campo y relación ancho/largo					
			20 cm^2			200 cm^2		
kV	mm Al	mm Cu	1:1	1:2	1:4	1:1	1:2	1:4
15	0.045	–	5.3	5.2	5.0	10.5	10.2	10.0
20	0.11	–	6.7	6.5	6.4	12.8	12.4	12.0
30	0.36	–	10.3	10.0	9.6	17.5	16.8	16.0
40	0.8	–	13.5	12.8	12.5	22	20.8	19.5
60	2.7	0.07	18.0	16.5	17.0	29	28	27
80	5.5	0.16	21	19.5	19.0	35	33	32
100	8	0.3	22	21	20	39	37	36
150	–	0.9	22	21	20	42	40	38
200	–	1.5	18.5	17.2	16.5	39	37	35
300	–	3.8	11.5	11.0	10.6	27	25	24
400	–	5.5	8.3	7.8	7.4	19.6	18.4	17.8
600	–	7.8	4.8	4.6	4.4	13.0	12.2	11.5
800	–	9	3.3	3.1	2.8	9.6	9.1	8.6
1000	–	10	2.5	2.3	2.1	7.8	7.4	7.0
Cs 137	–	–	1.7	1.5	1.3	6.0	5.5	5.3
2000	–	–	1.2	1.2	1.1	4.5	4.2	3.8
Co 60	–	–	1.1	1.1	1.1	3.9	3.8	3.4
3000	–	–	1.0	1.0	1.0	3.7	3.5	3.3

Lit.: 1. MAYNEORD, W.V., LAMERTON, L.F.: Brit.Radiol. 14, 255 (1941)
2. JOHNS, H.E.: Brit.J.Radiol. 25, 369 (1952)
3. JOHNS, H.E.: Physics of Radiation Therapy, Springfield: C.C. Thomas 1971
4. COHEN, M., JONES, D.E.A.: Brit.J.Radiol., Suppl. 11 (1972)

5.1.3 Variation of back scatter with body thickness (d)
Rückstreuung bei verschiedener Dicke des Streukörpers (d)
Variation de la rétrodiffusion en fonction de l'épaisseur (d)
Retrodispersión para diferentes espesores del fantoma (d)

100 cm^2 Field size - Feld - Champ - Campo

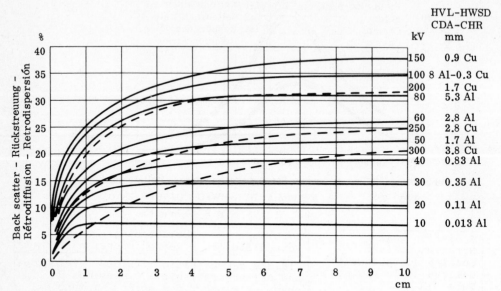

Body thickness - Körperdicke - Epaisseur du milieu - Espesor del cuerpo

d	Back scatter - Rückstreuung - Rétrodiffusion - Retrodispersión											%
	Radiation quality (normal radiation) - Strahlenqualität (Normalstrahlung) - Qualité du rayonnement (rayonnement normal) - Calidad de la radiación (radiación normal)											kV
cm	10	20	30	40	50	60	80	100	150	200	250	300
0.5	5.7	7.2	8.6	10	12	13	16	19	21	15	9.4	3.3
1	7.0	9.7	12	13	16	17	21	23	25	20	12	6.0
1.5	7.0	10	13	15	18	21	24	26	28	23	15	8.0
2	7.0	11	14	17	19	21	26	28	30	25	17	10
3	7.0	11	15	18	20	23	29	31	33	28	19	13
4	7.0	11	15	18	21	24	30	33	35	30	21	15
5	7.0	11	15	19	22	25	31	34	36	30	23	17
6	7.0	11	15	19	22	25	31	35	37	31	23	18
7	7.0	11	15	20	22	26	31	35	38	31	24	19
8	7.0	11	15	20	22	26	31	35	38	32	24	20
9	7.0	11	15	20	22	26	31	35	38	32	24	21
10	7.0	11	15	20	22	26	31	35	38	32	25	21

Lit.: 1. WACHSMANN, F., HECKEL, K., SCHIRREN, C.G.: Strahlenther. **94**, 161 (1954)

5.2 Half-value depth (HVD) of X- and gamma rays in tissue
Gewebehalbwerttiefen (GHWT) von Röntgen- und Gammastrahlen
Profondeur demi attenuation (PDA 50 %) dans les tissus pour
des rayonnements X et γ
Profundidades hemireductoras (PHR) para rayos X y γ
expresadas en espesor de tejido

5.2.1 Low energy X-rays - Weiche Röntgenstrahlen - Rayons X mous -
Rayos X blandos

0.1 - 8 mm Al HVL - HWSD - CDA - CHR

100 cm² Field size - Feldgröße - Champ - Campo

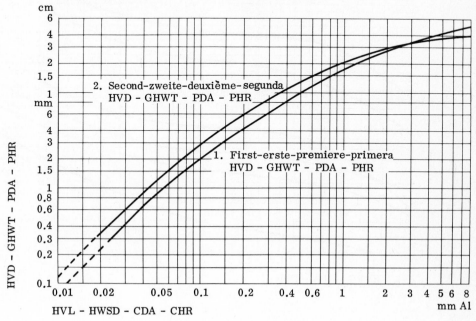

HVL - HWSD - CDA - CHR

HVL–HWSD CDA–CHR	HVD – GHWT PDA – PHR		HVL–HWSD CDA–CHR	HVD – GHWT PDA – PHR		HVL–HWSD CDA–CHR	HVD – GHWT PDA – PHR	
	1.	2.		1.	2.		1.	2.
mm Al	mm	mm	mm Al	mm	mm	mm Al	cm	cm
0.01	–	(0.12)	0.1	2.0	2.9	1	1.8	2.1
0.015	(0.15)	(0.22)	0.15	3.2	4.5	1.5	2.3	2.7
0.02	(0.23)	0.34	0.2	4.2	6.0	2	2.8	2.9
0.03	0.43	0.6	0.3	6.3	8.6	3	3.4	3.4
0.04	0.66	0.9	0.4	8.2	11	4	3.7	3.9
0.05	0.88	1.2	0.5	10	13	5	3.8	4.4
0.06	1.2	1.6	0.6	12	15	6	3.9	4.6
0.07	1.4	1.8	0.7	14	17	7	3.9	5.0
0.08	1.6	2.2	0.8	15	18	8	4.0	5.2
0.09	1.8	2.5	0.9	17	19			

Lit.: See pages - Siehe Seiten - Voir pages - Ver páginas 104 - 111

5.2.2 Orthovoltage X-rays - Harte Röntgenstrahlen - Rayons X classiques - Rayos X duros

0.5 - 8 mm Cu HVL - HWSD - CDA - CHR

50 cm FSD - FHA - DFP - DFP

25 - 100 - 200 cm^2 Field size - Feldgröße - Champ - Campo

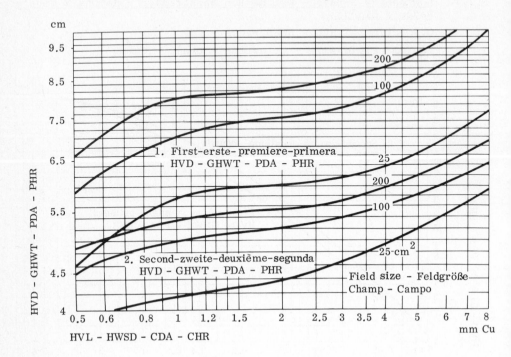

HVL-HWSD CDA-CHR	HVD - GHWT PDA - PHR (100 cm^2)		HVL-HWSD CDA-CHR	HVD - GHWT PDA - PHR (100 cm^2)	
	1.	2.		1.	2.
mm Cu	cm	cm	mm Cu	cm	cm
0.5	5.9	4.5	2	7.5	5.2
0.6	6.3	4.7	2.5	7.6	5.3
0.7	6.5	4.8	3	7.7	5.4
0.8	6.7	4.9	3.5	7.9	5.5
0.9	6.9	4.9	4	8.1	5.6
1	7.0	5.0	4.5	8.3	5.7
1.1	7.1	5.0	5	8.5	5.8
1.2	7.2	5.1	5.5	8.8	5.9
1.3	7.3	5.1	6	9.0	6.0
1.4	7.3	5.1	7	9.4	6.2
1.5	7.4	5.1	8	10	6.4

Lit.: See pages - Siehe Seiten - Voir pages - Ver paginas 87 - 99

5.2.3   <u>Super- and megavoltage X- and gamma rays</u>
        <u>Sehr harte und ultraharte Röntgen- und Gammastrahlen</u>
        <u>Rayons X de haute et très haute énergie et rayons gamma</u>
        <u>Rayos X muy duros, ultraduros y gamma</u>

0.5 - 100 MV

100 cm FSD - FHA - DFP - DFP

(50-) 100 (-200) cm^2 Field size - Feldgröße - Champ - Campo

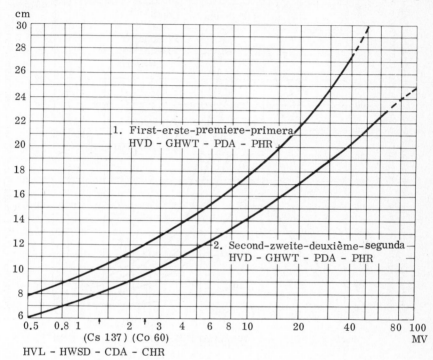

HVD - GHWT - PDA - PHR

1. First-erste-premiere-primera
   HVD - GHWT - PDA - PHR

2. Second-zweite-deuxième-segunda
   HVD - GHWT - PDA - PHR

(Cs 137) (Co 60)

HVL - HWSD - CDA - CHR

HVL–HWSD CDA–CHR	HVD – GHWT PDA – PHR (100 cm^2)		HVL–HWSD CDA–CHR	HVD – GHWT PDA – PHR (100 cm^2)	
	1.	2.		1.	2.
MeV	cm	cm	MeV	cm	cm
0.5	8.0	6.0	6	15.5	12.3
0.6	8.4	6.4	8	16.8	13.2
0.8	9.0	7.0	10	17.7	14.0
1	9.4	7.4	15	19.7	15.7
Cs 137	10.1	8.0	20	21.7	17.1
1.5	10.5	8.3	30	24.8	19.0
2	11.5	9.6	40	27.4	20.3
Co 60	12.1	9.7	50	(29.6)	21.4
3	12.5	10.3	60	–	22.4
4	13.8	11.1	80	–	(24.0)
5	14.5	11.7	100	–	(24.9)

Lit.: See pages-Siehe Seiten-Voir pages-Ver paginas 118-122, 126-129

5.3 Primary and scattered radiation at different depths
Primär- und Streustrahlung in verschiedenen Tiefen
Rayonnement primaire et diffusé à diverses profondeurs
Radiación primaria y dispersa a distintas profundidades

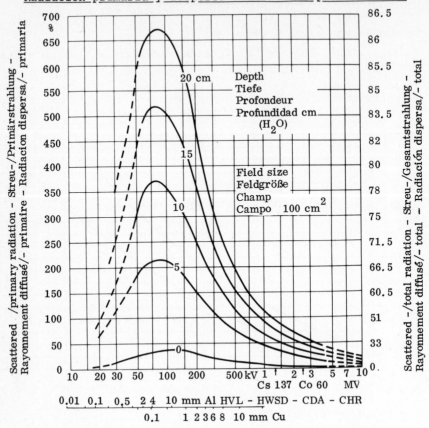

Tube voltage - Röhrenspannung - Tension d'alimentation
Tensión del tubo

In the case of larger or smaller fields the amount of scattered radiation increases or decreases, respectively, approximately with the square root of the field size.

Bei größeren bzw. kleineren Feldern wächst bzw. fällt der Streustrahlenanteil etwa mit der Quadratwurzel aus der Feldgröße.

Pour de plus grands ou de plus petits champs, la proportion du rayonnement diffusé augmente ou diminue à peu près avec la racine carrée de la dimension du champ.

En el caso de campos mayores o menores, la porción de radiación dispersada aumenta o disminuye aproximadamente con la raiz cuadrada de la magnitud del campo.

Lit.: 1. GAJEWSKI, H.: Fortschr. Röntgenstr. 80, 642 (1954)

Radiation quality Strahlenqualität Qualité du rayonnement Calidad de la radiación			Scattered/primary radiation Streu-/Primärstrahlung Rayonnement diffusé/- primaire Radiación dispersa/- primaria %				
	HVL - HWSD CDA - CHR		Depth-Tiefe-Profondeur-Profundidad cm				
kV-MV	mm		0	5	10	15	20
20 kV	0.11 Al		–	(52)	(95)	–	–
30 kV	0.35		12	(110)	(170)	(275)	(370)
40 kV	0.83		19	(150)	(240)	(360)	(480)
50 kV	1.7	0.045 Cu	25	190	300	(440)	(580)
60 kV	2.8	0.07	29	210	350	480	640
80 kV	5.3	0.16	34	215	370	520	670
100 kV	8.0	0.30	38	212	360	505	665
150 kV		0.9	35	180	305	440	590
200 kV		1.7	29	150	250	360	475
300 kV		3.8	21	110	175	240	315
400 kV		5.8	18	90	140	185	290
500 kV		7.1	14	75	115	158	200
600 kV		8.0	12	65	100	137	168
800 kV		9.0	9	55	80	110	135
1 MV		10	7	45	67	93	114
Cs 137		–	5	40	57	76	95
2 MV		–	4	28	42	55	70
Co 60		–	2	22	37	47	62
5 MV		–	(1)	(14)	(21)	(30)	(39)

Radiation quality Strahlenqualität Qualité du rayonnement Calidad de la raciación			Scattered /total radiation Streu-/Gesamtstrahlung Rayonnement diffusé/- total Radiación dispersa/- total %				
	HVL - HWSD CDA - CHR		Depth-Tiefe-Profondeur-Profundidad cm				
kV-MV	mm		0	5	10	15	20
20 kV	0.11 Al		–	(34)	(49)	–	–
30 kV	0.35		10	(52)	(63)	(73)	(78)
40 kV	0.83		16	(60)	(70)	(79)	(83)
50 kV	1.7	0.045 Cu	20	66	75	(82)	(86)
60 kV	2.8	0.07	22	67	78	83	86
80 kV	5.3	0.16	25	68	79	84	87
100 kV	8.0	0.30	27	68	78	83	86
150 kV		0.9	26	64	75	82	84
200 kV		1.7	23	60	72	78	83
300 kV		3.8	18	52	63	71	77
400 kV		5.8	15	47	58	65	75
500 kV		7.1	12	43	54	61	67
600 kV		8.0	10	40	50	57	63
800 kV		9.0	8	35	44	52	58
1 MV		10	6.5	31	40	48	53
Cs 137		–	4.7	28	36	43	49
2 MV		–	4.0	22	30	35	41
Co 60		–	2	18	28	32	38
5 MV		–	(1)	(12)	(17)	(23)	(28)

5.4 <u>Dose fall-off outside the beam axis (dose decrement)</u>
<u>Abfall der Dosis seitlich vom Zentralstrahl (Dosisdekrement)</u>
<u>Décroissance de la dose en traversée</u>
<u>Disminución de la dosis lateral del rayo central</u>

Values measured in a water phantom 80 x 40 x 30 cm for 50 cm FSD -
In einem Wasserphantom von 80 x 40 x 30 cm gemessene Werte bei 50 cm
FHA - Valeurs mesurées dans un fantôme d'eau de 80 x 40 x 30 cm, DSP
50 cm - Valores medidos en un fantoma de agua de 80 x 40 x 30 cm a
50 cm DFP

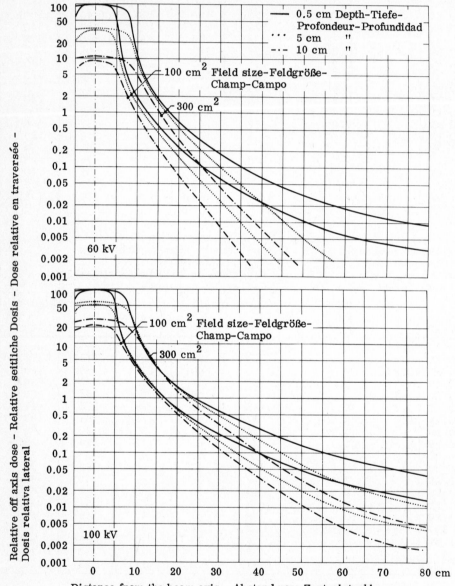

Distance from the beam axis - Abstand vom Zentralstrahl -
Distance de l'axe du faisceau - Distancia del rayo central

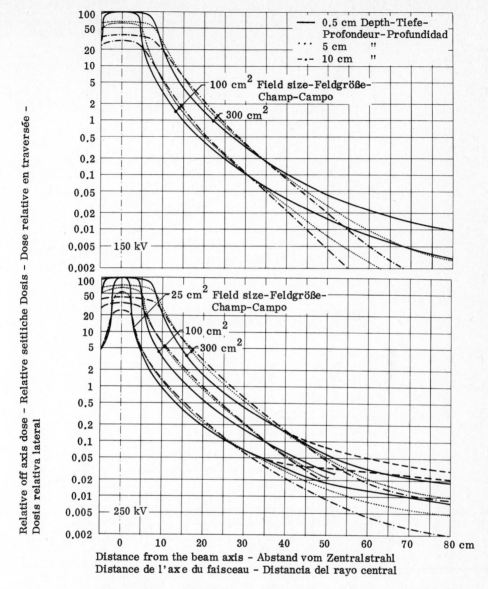

Relative off axis dose – Relative seitliche Dosis – Dose relative en traversée – Dosis relativa lateral

Distance from the beam axis - Abstand vom Zentralstrahl
Distance de l'axe du faisceau - Distancia del rayo central

--- Dose at 0.5 cm depth including the radiation passing through the tube housing (Siemens therapy tube housing Z Rhb 2, 250 kV)

--- Dosis in 0,5 cm Tiefe einschließlich der Gehäusedurchlaßstrahlung (Siemens Therapiehaube Z Rhb 2, 250 kV)

--- Dose à 0,5 cm de profondeur incluant la dose dûe au rayonnement de fuite à travers de la gaine du tube (gaine de thérapie Siemens Z Rhb 2, 250 kV)

--- Dosis a una profundidad de 0,5 cm incluida la radiación a través de la carcasa del tubo (carcasa para la terapía, Siemens Z Rhb 2, 250 kV)

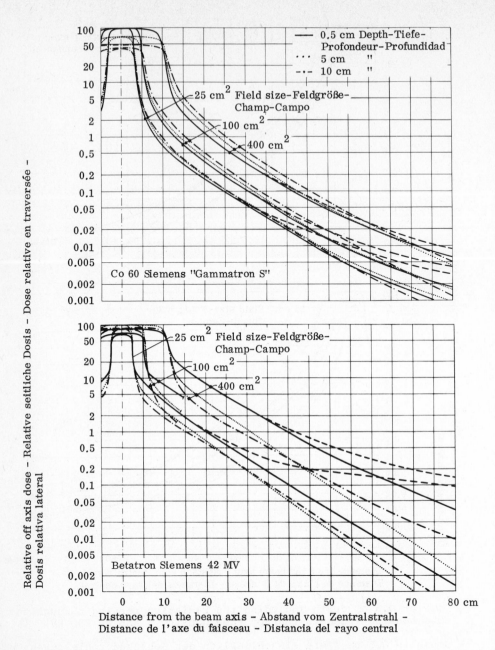

Relative off axis dose - Relative seitliche Dosis - Dose relative en traversée -
Dosis relativa lateral

— 0.5 cm Depth-Tiefe-
Profondeur-Profundidad
··· 5 cm "
—·— 10 cm "

25 cm^2 Field size-Feldgröße-
Champ-Campo

100 cm^2

400 cm^2

Co 60 Siemens "Gammatron S"

25 cm^2 Field size-Feldgröße-
Champ-Campo

100 cm^2

400 cm^2

Betatron Siemens 42 MV

Distance from the beam axis - Abstand vom Zentralstrahl -
Distance de l'axe du faisceau - Distancia del rayo central

--- See page - Siehe Seite - Voir page - Ver página 147

Lit.: 1. SEELENTAG, W., KLOTZ E.: Strahlenther. 108, 112 (1959)
      2. WACHSMANN, F., JASCHKE, R.: Biophysik 1, 108 (1963)
      3. TROUT, D.E., KELLEY, J.P.: Am.J.Roentgenol. 85, 546 (1965)
      4. CZEMPIEL, H., MÜHLE, P., REGULLA, D.F., WACHSMANN, F.:
         Fortschr.Röntgenstr. 124, (1976) im Druck

Table of contents - Inhaltsverzeichnis
Table des matières - Tabla de materias

6.1 Radionuclides used in nuclear medicine
In der Nuklearmedizin verwendete Radionuklide
Radionucleides utilisés en médecine nucléaire
Radionuclidos utilizados en medicina nuclear

Nuclide Nuklid Nucléide Nuclido	$T_{1/2}$	Decay Zerfall Décroissance Desintegr.	E_β max. MeV	E_γ max. MeV	P_γ %	Γ $R\ \dfrac{m^2}{Ci\ h}$	Appl.
^3H, T	12.3 a	β^-	0.0186	–	–	–	D,R,T
^{14}C	5700 a	β^-	0.156	–	–	–	D,R,T
^{13}N	10 min	β^+	1.2	0.511	200	0.59	D
^{18}F	110 min	β^+,EC	0.64	0.511	190	0.57	D,R
^{22}Na	2.6 a	β^+,EC	0.54 1.8	0.511 1.27	180 200	1.19	D
^{24}Na	15 h	β^-	1.39	1.37 2.75	100 100	1.82	D
^{32}P	14.3 d	β^-	1.71	–	–	–	D,Th
^{35}S	88 d	β^-	0.167	–	–	–	D
^{40}K	$1.28 \cdot 10^9$ a	β^-,EC	1.32	1.46	11	0.0803	R
^{42}K	12.4 h	β^-	3.52	1.52	18	0.137	D
^{45}Ca	165 d	β^-	0.252	–	–	–	D,R
^{47}Ca	4.53 d	β^-	0.67 1.98	0.5 0.81 1.3	5 5 74	– 0.54	D
^{51}Cr	27.8 d	E		0.32	9	0.018	D
^{52}Fe	8 h	β^+,EC	0.80	0.17 0.511	100 112	0.41	D
^{55}Fe	2.6 a	EC	–	0.006*)		–	D
^{59}Fe	45 d	β^-	0.48	0.19 1.1 1.29	3 56 44	0.62	D
^{57}Co	269 d	EC	–	0.006*) 0.014 0.12 0.14	9 87 11	0.093	D
^{58}Co	713 d	β^+,EC	0.47	0.006*) 0.511 0.81	30 99	0.54	D
^{60}Co	5.27 a	β^-	0.31	1.17 1.33	100 100	1.30	Th,T D,R
^{64}Cu	12.8 h	β^-,EC β^-	0.66 0.57	0.008*) 0.511 –	38 –	0.116 –	D
^{65}Zn	246 d	β^+	0.33	0.511 1.12	3 49	0.30	D

Nuclide Nuklid Nucléide Nuclido	$T_{1/2}$	Decay Zerfall Décroissance Desintegr.	Energy-Energie Energie-Energia		P_γ %	$\dfrac{\Gamma}{R \dfrac{m^2}{Ci\ h}}$	Appl.
			E_β max. MeV	E_γ max. MeV			
^{68}Ga	68 min	β^+,EC	1.9	0.009*) 0.511 1.08	176 4	0.54	D
^{72}Ga	14.2 h	β^-	3.1	0.60 0.63 0.84 0.89 2.2 2.5	8 27 96 10 26 20	1.31	D,R
^{68}Ge	275 d	EC	–	0.009*)		–	D,R
^{74}As	17.7 d	β^+,EC β^+ β^-	0.95 1.5 1.4	0.01*) 0.511 0.6 0.64	59 61 14	0.45	D
^{76}As	26.4 h	β^-	2.97	0.56 0.66 1.22	43 6 5	0.25	D,R
^{75}Se	122 d	EC	–	0.011*) 0.12 0.14 0.26 0.28 0.4	17 57 60 25 12	0.20	D,R
^{85}Kr	10.2 a	β^-	0.67	0.51	4	0.0012	D,T
^{86}Rb	18.7 d	β^-	1.78	1.08	9	0.051	D
^{87}Rb	$4.8 \cdot 10^{10}$a	β^-	0.27	–		–	D
^{85}Sr	64.7 d	EC	–	0.014*) 0.511	100	0.30	D
^{87m}Sr	2.8 h	–	0.37 e 0.39 e	0.39	80	0.18	D
^{89}Sr	53 d	β^-	1.46	–	–	–	D,R
^{90}Sr	28 a	β^-	0.55	–	–	–	Th,T
^{90}Y	64 h	β^-	2.27	–	–	–	Th
^{99}Mo	66.5 h	β^-	1.23	0.04 0.18 0.37 0.74 0.78	2 7 1 12 4	0.83	D,R
^{99m}Tc	6.0 h		0.12 e	0.14	90	0.061	D
^{111}Ag	7.4 d	β^-	1.05	0.25 0.34	1 6	0.013	D
^{113m}In	102 min		0.36 e 0.39 e	0.39	64	0.145	D
^{113}Sn	120 d	EC	–	0.015*) 0.25	1.8	0.003	D,R

Nuclide Nuklid Nucléide Nuclido	$T_{1/2}$	Decay Zerfall Décroissance Desintegr.	Energy-Energie Energie-Energîa $E_\beta$max. MeV	$E_\gamma$max. MeV	P_γ %	$\frac{\Gamma}{R \frac{m^2}{Ci\ h}}$	Appl.
^{132}Te	77.8 h	β^-	0.22	0.05	17		
				0.23	90	0.121	D,R
^{123}I^{123}J	13.1 h	EC	–	0.028*)			
				0.16	83	0.072	R
^{125}I^{125}J	59.2 d	EC	–	0.028*)			
				0.035	7	0.004	D
^{128}I^{128}J	25 min	β^-,EC	2.12	0.028*)			
				0.441	14	0.053	D
^{131}I^{131}J	8.07 d	β^-	0.61	0.08	3		
				0.28	5	0.21	D,Th
			0.81	0.36	82		
				0.64	7		
^{132}I^{132}J	2.35 h	β^-	2.1	0.52	20		
				0.67	144		
				0.77	89		
				0.96	22	1.13	D,Th
				1.14	6		
				1.28	7		
				1.4	14		
^{133}Xe	5.4 d	β^-	0.35	0.08	37	0.014	D
^{137}Cs	30 a	β^-	0.51	0.662	85	0.323	Th,T
			1.18				
^{170}Tm	129 d	β^-	0.97	0.084	3.3	0.001	D,R
^{182}Ta	115 d	β^-	0.52	0.07	42		
				0.1	14		
			1.71	0.15	7		
				0.22	8	0.68	Th
				1.12	34		
				1.19	16		
				1.22	27		
				1.23	13		
^{192}Ir	74.3 d	β^-,EC	0.67	0.3	29		
				0.31	30		
				0.32	81		
				0.47	49	0.51	Th,T
				0.59	4		
				0.6	9		
				0.61	6		
^{198}Au	2.7 d	β^-	0.96	0.41	95		
				0.68	1	0.233	D,Th
^{199}Au	3.15 d	β^-	0.3	0.16	37		
			0.46	0.21	8	0.078	R,Th
^{197}Hg	65 h	EC	–	0.071*)		0.009	D
				0.08	18		
				0.19	2		
^{203}Hg	47.1 d	β^-	0.21	0.28	77	0.175	D

Nuclide Nuklid Nucléide Nuclido	$T_{1/2}$	Decay Zerfall Décroissance Desintegr.	Energy-Energie Energie-Energía $E_{\beta,\alpha}$ MeV	E_γ max. MeV	P_γ %	Γ $\dfrac{R\ m^2}{Ci\ h}$	Appl.
^{206}Bi	6.24 d	EC		0.077*) 0.52 0.8 0.88 1.7	46 99 72 36	1.86	Th,D
^{222}Rn	3.82 d	α	5.49				R,Th
^{224}Ra	3.64 d	α	5.45	0.24	4	0.005	T,Th
^{226}Ra	1600 a	α	4.78	0.186	4	0.004 0.83**)	T,Th
^{228}Th	1.91 a	α	5.34 5.43	0.084	2	0.007	T
^{230}Th	$7.9\cdot10^4$a	α	4.62 4.68	0.068	0.6	0.0003	T,R
^{232}T	$1.4\cdot10^{10}$a	α	3.9 4.0				R,T
^{235}U	$7\cdot10^8$a	α	4.37 4.40 4.58	0.11 0.14 0.16 0.18 0.2	2.5 11 5 54 6	0.071	T
^{238}U	$4.5\cdot10^9$a	α	4.15 4.20				T
^{239}Pu	$2.4\cdot10^4$a	α	5.11 5.16	0.013 0.038 0.051	17	0.02	T
^{252}Cf	2.2 a	α	6.12 6.08	0.043 0.1 0.160			Th
^{252}Cf	85 a	n	2.13				

P_γ: Emission probability (% of disintegrations) - Emissionswahr-
scheinlichkeit (% der Zerfälle) - Probabilité d'émission (%
du nombre de desintégrations) - Probabilidad de emisiòn (% de
desintegración)

Γ: Specific gamma-ray constant - Spezifische Gammastrahlenkon-
stante - Constante de débit d'exposition - Constante específica de radiación gamma

Appl.: Application - Anwendung - Utilisation - Aplicación

D: Diagnosis; Th: Therapy; R: Research; T: Technology

e: Conversion electrons - Konversionselektronen - Conversion
interne - Electrones de conversión

EC: Electron capture - Elektroneneinfang - Capture électronique -
Captura de electrones

*) K-radiation - K-Strahlung - Rayonnement K - Radiación K
**) Ra 226 + decay products - Ra 226 + Zerfallsprodukte - Ra 226 +
produits de désintegration - Ra 226+ productos de desintegración

6.2 Desintegration schemes of radionuclides
Zerfallsschemen von Radionukliden
Schémas de désintégration des radionucléides
Esquemas de desintegración de radionúclidos

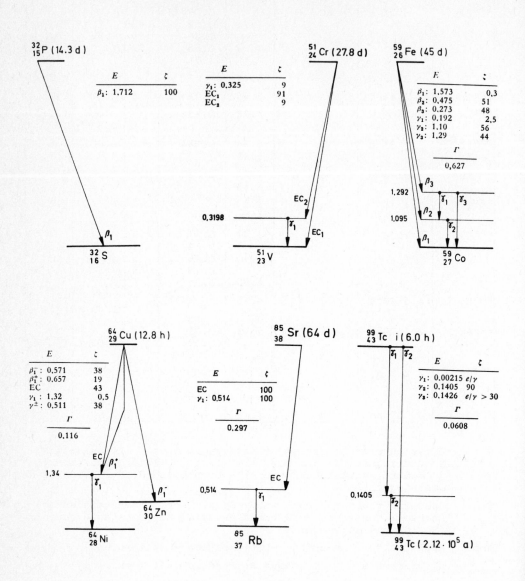

Lit.: 1. LEDERER, C.M., HOLLANDER, J.M., PERLMAN, J.: Table of Iso-
        topes, New York: J. Wiley & Sons, Inc. 1967

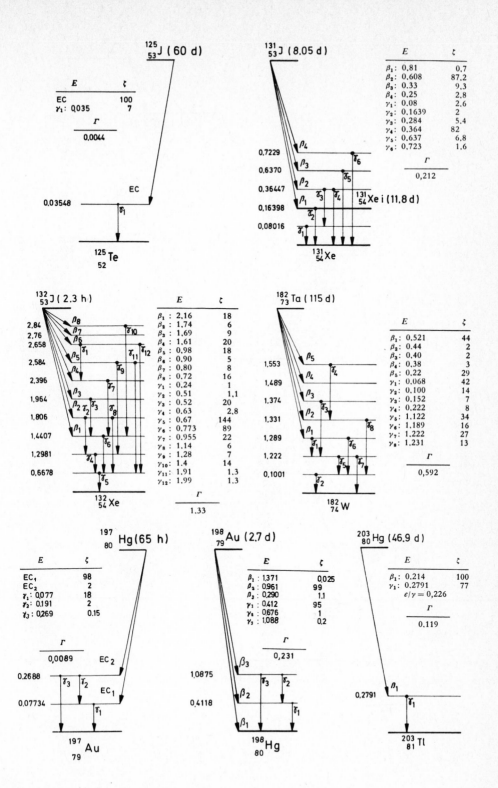

$^{125}_{53}\text{J}$ (60 d)

E	ζ
EC	100
γ₁: 0,035	7

Γ

0,0044

EC

0,03548

γ₁

$^{125}_{52}\text{Te}$

$^{131}_{53}\text{J}$ (8,05 d)

E	ζ
β₁: 0,81	0,7
β₂: 0,608	87,2
β₃: 0,33	9,3
β₄: 0,25	2,8
γ₁: 0,08	2,6
γ₂: 0,1639	2
γ₃: 0,284	5,4
γ₄: 0,364	82
γ₅: 0,637	6,8
γ₆: 0,723	1,6

Γ

0,212

0,7229   β₄   γ₆
0,6370   β₃   γ₅
0,36447   β₂
0,16398   β₁   γ₃ γ₄ $^{131}_{54}\text{Xe i}$ (11,8 d)
          γ₂
0,08016
          γ₁

$^{131}_{54}\text{Xe}$

$^{132}_{53}\text{J}$ (2,3 h)

E	ζ
β₁ : 2,16	18
β₂ : 1,74	6
β₃ : 1,69	9
β₄ : 1,61	20
β₅ : 0,98	18
β₆ : 0,90	5
β₇ : 0,80	8
β₈ : 0,72	16
γ₁ : 0,24	1
γ₂ : 0,51	1,1
γ₃ : 0,52	20
γ₄ : 0,63	2,8
γ₅ : 0,67	144
γ₆ : 0,773	89
γ₇ : 0,955	22
γ₈ : 1,14	6
γ₉ : 1,28	7
γ₁₀: 1,4	14
γ₁₁: 1,91	1,3
γ₁₂: 1,99	1,3

Γ

1.33

2,84   β₈   γ₁₀
2,76   β₇
2,658   β₆
          γ₁   γ₁₁ γ₁₂
2,584   β₅
                   γ₉
2,396   β₄
          γ₇
1,964   β₃
          β₂ γ₂ γ₃   γ₈
1,806   β₁
1,4407   γ₆
1,2981   γ₄
0,6678   γ₅

$^{132}_{54}\text{Xe}$

$^{182}_{73}\text{Ta}$ (115 d)

E	ζ
β₁: 0,521	44
β₂: 0,44	2
β₃: 0,40	2
β₄: 0,38	3
β₅: 0,22	29
γ₁: 0,068	42
γ₂: 0,100	14
γ₃: 0,152	7
γ₄: 0,222	8
γ₅: 1,122	34
γ₆: 1,189	16
γ₇: 1,222	27
γ₈: 1,231	13

Γ

0,592

1,553   β₅   γ₄
1,489   β₄
1,374   β₃
1,331   β₂   γ₃
1,289   β₁   γ₈
1,222   γ₁   γ₆
          γ₁   γ₅ γ₇
0,1001
          γ₂

$^{182}_{74}\text{W}$

$^{197}_{80}\text{Hg}$ (65 h)

E	ζ
EC₁	98
EC₂	2
γ₁: 0,077	18
γ₂: 0,191	2
γ₃: 0,269	0,15

Γ

0,0089   EC₂

0,2688   γ₃ γ₂   EC₁

0,07734   γ₁

$^{197}_{79}\text{Au}$

$^{198}_{79}\text{Au}$ (2,7 d)

E	ζ
β₁ : 1,371	0,025
β₂ : 0,961	99
β₃ : 0,290	1,1
γ₁ : 0,412	95
γ₂ : 0,676	1
γ₃ : 1,088	0,2

Γ

0,231

β₃

1,0875   β₂   γ₃ γ₂

0,4118   β₁   γ₁

$^{198}_{80}\text{Hg}$

$^{203}_{80}\text{Hg}$ (46,9 d)

E	ζ
β₁: 0,214	100
γ₁: 0,2791	77
e/γ = 0,226	

Γ

0,119

0,2791   β₁   γ₁

$^{203}_{81}\text{Tl}$

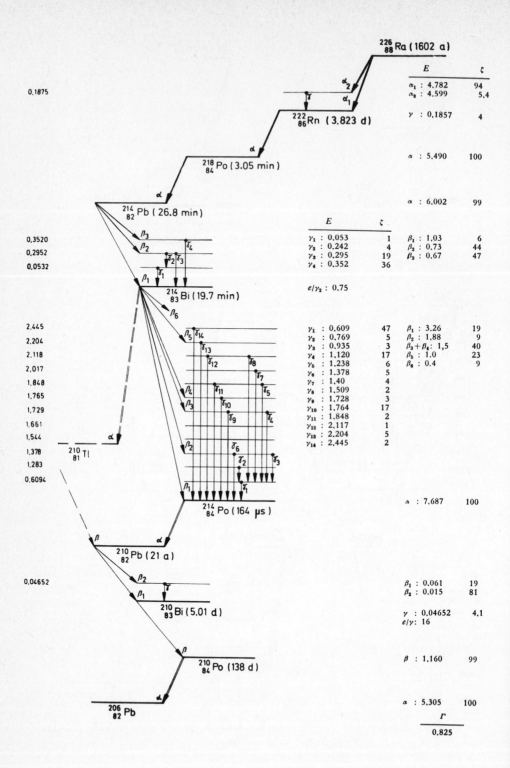

0.1875

$^{226}_{88}$Ra (1602 a)

$^{222}_{86}$Rn (3.823 d)

$^{218}_{84}$Po (3.05 min)

α_2
α_1

E	ζ
α_1 : 4.782	94
α_2 : 4.599	5,4
γ : 0.1857	4
α : 5.490	100
α : 6.002	99

$^{214}_{82}$Pb (26.8 min)

0.3520 β_3
0.2952 β_2
0.0532 β_1

$^{214}_{83}$Bi (19.7 min)

E	ζ
γ_1 : 0.053	1
γ_2 : 0.242	4
γ_3 : 0.295	19
γ_4 : 0.352	36

e/γ_2 : 0.75

β_1 : 1.03	6
β_2 : 0.73	44
β_3 : 0.67	47

β_6

2.445
2.204
2.118
2.017
1.848
1.765
1.729
1.661
1.544
1.378 $^{210}_{81}$Tl
1.283
0.6094

α

γ_1 : 0.609	47	β_1 : 3.26	19
γ_2 : 0.769	5	β_2 : 1.88	9
γ_3 : 0.935	3	$\beta_3+\beta_4$: 1,5	40
γ_4 : 1.120	17	β_5 : 1.0	23
γ_5 : 1.238	6	β_6 : 0.4	9
γ_6 : 1.378	5		
γ_7 : 1.40	4		
γ_8 : 1.509	2		
γ_9 : 1.728	3		
γ_{10} : 1.764	17		
γ_{11} : 1.848	2		
γ_{12} : 2.117	1		
γ_{13} : 2.204	5		
γ_{14} : 2.445	2		

$^{214}_{84}$Po (164 μs)

α : 7.687   100

$^{210}_{82}$Pb (21 a)

0.04652 β_2
β_1

$^{210}_{83}$Bi (5.01 d)

β_1 : 0.061	19
β_2 : 0.015	81

γ : 0.04652   4,1
e/γ: 16

$^{210}_{84}$Po (138 d)

β : 1.160   99

$^{206}_{82}$Pb

α : 5.305   100

Γ

0.825

6.3 <u>Exposure rates of radium and other radionuclides at different distances from point sources given in Ci and Bq</u>

<u>Dosisleistung von Radium und anderen Radionukliden in verschiedenen Abständen von punktförmigen Quellen in Ci und Bq</u>

<u>Débit d'exposition pour le radium et autres radionucléides à diverses distances de sources ponctuelles en Ci et Bq</u>

<u>Potencia de dosis del radio y otros radionúclidos a diferentes distancias de fuentes puntiformes expresado en Ci y Bq</u>

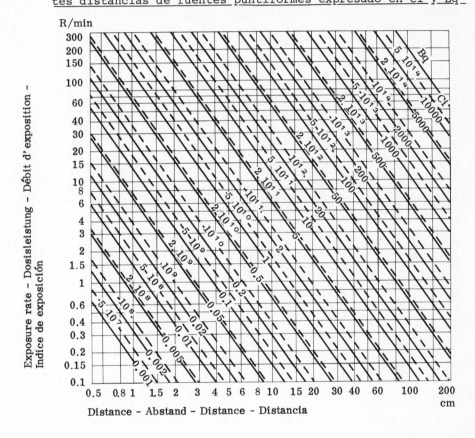

Distance - Abstand - Distance - Distancia

The exposure rates of radium sources filtered with 0.5 mm Pt; self-absorption in the source is disregarded.

Dosisleistungen von Radium bei einer Filterung von 0,5 mm Pt ohne Berücksichtigung der Selbstabsorption in der Quelle.

Les débits d'exposition sont donnés pour le radium filtré par 0.5 mm Pt; on n'a pas tenu compte de l'autoabsorption dans la source.

Las potencias de las dosis indicadas están referidas al radio filtrado con 0,5 mm Pt, despreciando la autoabsorción en la fuente.

Activity Aktivität Activité Actividad	Exposure rate of Ra 226 at various distances - Dosisleistung von Ra 226 in verschiedenen Abständen - Débit d'exposition de Ra 226 à diverses distances - Potencia de la dosis de Ra 226 a varias distancias R/min								
	Distance - Abstand - Distance - Distancia cm								
Ci	1	1.5	2	2.5	3	4	5	6	8
1	138	61.5	34.5	22.1	15.3	8.6	5.5	3.83	2.15
1.2	166	73.8	41.5	26.5	18.4	10.4	6.6	4.60	2.57
1.4	194	86.0	48.4	31.0	21.4	12.1	7.7	5.3	3.00
1.6	221	98.5	55.3	35.4	24.5	13.8	8.8	6.1	3.45
1.8	249	110	62.3	39.8	27.5	16.6	9.9	6.9	3.87
2	276	124	69	44.2	30.6	17.2	11.0	7.7	4.3
2.5	345	154	86.4	55.2	38.3	21.6	13.8	9.6	5.4
3	415	185	104	66.5	46.0	25.9	16.5	11.5	6.5
3.5	484	216	121	77.5	53.6	30.2	19.2	13.4	7.5
4	552	247	138	88.6	61.2	34.4	22.0	15.3	8.6
4.5	622	277	155	99.6	68.8	38.8	24.8	17.2	9.6
5	690	308	172	111	76.6	43.2	27.5	19.2	10.8
6	830	370	207	133	92.0	51.8	33.0	23.0	12.9
7	970	432	242	155	107	60.4	38.5	26.8	15.1
8	1104	493	276	177	122	68.8	44.0	30.6	17.2
9	2242	554	310	199	138	77.8	49.5	34.5	19.4
TBq	1	1.5	2	2.5	3	4	5	6	8
1	37.2	16.5	9.3	6.0	4.1	2.32	1.48	1.03	0.58
1.2	44.8	19.8	11.2	7.2	5.0	2.78	1.77	1.23	0.70
1.4	52.1	23.1	13.0	8.4	5.8	3.25	2.07	1.44	0.81
1.6	59.7	26.5	14.9	9.6	6.6	3.72	2.37	1.64	0.93
1.8	67.2	29.7	16.8	10.8	7.5	4.17	2.67	1.85	1.04
2	74.4	33.0	18.6	12.0	8.3	4.65	2.95	2.05	1.16
2.5	93.0	41.3	23.3	15.0	10.4	5.8	3.70	2.56	1.45
3	111	49.5	27.9	18.0	12.4	6.7	4.45	3.08	1.74
3.5	130	57.8	32.5	21.0	14.5	8.1	5.2	3.60	2.04
4	148	66.1	37.2	24.0	16.5	9.3	5.9	4.10	2.32
4.5	167	74.4	41.9	27.0	18.6	10.5	6.7	4.60	2.62
5	185	82.8	46.5	30.0	20.6	11.6	7.4	5.1	2.90
6	222	99.0	55.8	36.0	24.8	14.0	8.9	6.2	3.48
7	259	116	65.1	42.0	28.9	16.2	10.4	7.2	4.05
8	296	132	74.5	48.0	33.0	18.6	11.8	8.2	4.65
9	334	148	83.8	54.0	27.1	20.9	13.3	9.2	5.2

For activities other than those listed in the table, the exposure rates can easily be calculated in direct proportion to the activity and in inverse proportion to the square of the distance by means of decimal factors.

Für andere als in der Tabelle angegebene Aktivitäten lassen sich die Dosisleistungen proportional der Aktivität und umgekehrt proportional dem Quadrat des Abstandes unter Verwendung dekadischer Multiplikationsfaktoren leicht berechnen.

Pour des activités autres que celles figurant dans la table, les débits d'exposition peuvent facilement être calculés en proportion directe de l'activité et en proportion inverse du carré de la distance.

Actividades diferentes a las que aparecen en la tabla se pueden calcular facilmente mediante proporción directa de la actividad y proporción inversa del cuadrado de la distancia utilizando factores de multiplicación decimales.

The exposure rates for other radionuclides than Ra 226 can be calculated by multiplication of the values from the curve or the table by
the following values which correspond to the relationship of specific gamma ray constants ($\Gamma_x/\Gamma_{Ra\ 226}$).

Die Dosisleistungen anderer Radionuklide als Ra 226 ergeben sich
durch Multiplikation der aus den Kurven oder aus der Tabelle entnom-
menen Werten mit folgenden, dem Verhältnis der spezifischen Gamma-
strahlenkonstanten entsprechenden, Werten ($\Gamma_x/\Gamma_{Ra\ 226}$).

Les débits d'exposition pour d'autres radionucléides que Ra 226
peuvent être calculés en multipliant les valeurs des courbes où de
la table par les facteurs suivants de débit d'exposition
($\Gamma_x/\Gamma_{Ra\ 226}$).

La potencia de la dosis de otros radionúclidos del que Ra 226 se
puede calcular multiplicando los valores des las curvas o de la
tabla por los siguientes valores que corresponden a las relaciones
de las constantes específicas de rayos gamma ($\Gamma_x/\Gamma_{Ra\ 226}$).

Specific γ-ray constants - Spezifische γ-Strahlenkonstanten - Facteurs specifiques de rayons γ - Constantes especificas de rayos γ Γ					
^{46}Sc	^{60}Co	^{110}Ag	^{131}I	^{137}Cs	^{144}Ce
1.32	1.58	1.80	0.255	0.39	0.03
^{154}Eu	^{160}Tb	^{170}Tm	^{182}Ta	^{192}Ir	^{198}Au
0.78	0.98	0.0012	0.83	0.62	0.283

The self-absorption which, for Co 60, amounts to about 10 % per cm
of source height and for Cs 137, to about 15 % per g/cm^2, is diffi-
cult to calculate because the packing density of the radioactive
material is usually unknown. Therefore, the activity of large sources presently is expressed not in Ci, but directly in R/h at a 1 m
distance in free air, or preferably in water at 5 cm depth.

Die Selbstabsorption, die bei Co 60 etwa 10 % je cm Quellenhöhe und
bei Cs 137 etwa 15 % der g/cm^2 beträgt, läßt sich wegen der meist
unbekannten Packungsdichte des radioaktiven Materials schwer berechnen. Deshalb wird die Stärke von Großquellen heute nicht in Ci son-
dern direkt in R/h in 1 m Abstand frei in Luft oder besser in 5 cm
Wassertiefe angegeben.

L'auto-absorption qui s'élève à environ 10 % par cm de hauteur pour
les sources de Co 60 et à 15 % par g/cm^2 pour le Cs 137 est diffi-
cile à calculer car la densité réelle du matériau radioactif est
habituellement inconnue. C'est pourqoi l'activité des grandes sourses
est actuellement exprimée ne pas en Ci, mais directement en R/h à
une distance de 1 m, dans l'air, ou de préférence à une profondeur
de 5 cm dans l'eau.

La autoabsorción, que para el Co 60 supone aproximadamente el 10 %
por cm de altura de la fuente y para el Cs 137 aproximadamente el
15 % por g/cm^2, se puede calcular dificilmente debido a que generalmente no se conoce la densidad de empaquetamiento del material radioactivo. Por esta razón la intensidad de fuentes grandes no se mide
hoy en Ci sino en R/h a 1 m de distancia en aire o mejor a 5 cm de
profundidad de agua.

6.4 Decay of the activity of radionuclides with time
Abnahme der Aktivität von Radionukliden mit der Zeit
Décroissance de l'activité des radionucléides avec le temps
Disminución de la actividad de radionúclidos con el tiempo

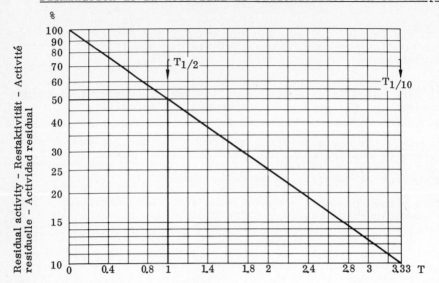

Time - Zeit - Temps - Tiempo

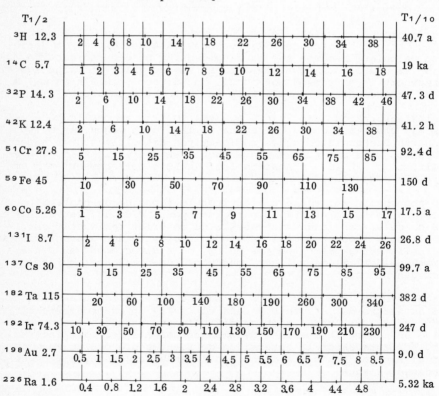

6.4.1   Time required to reach a given residual activity
Zeit zum Erreichen einer bestimmten Restaktivität
Temps nécessaire pour atteindre une activité résiduelle
Tiempo necesario para alcanzar una actividad residual

Nuclide Nuklid Nucléide Nuclido	Time - Zeit - Temps - Tiempo									h, d, a, ka
	Residual activity - Restaktivität - Activité résiduelle - Actividad residual %									
	90	80	70	60	50	40	30	25	20	10
^{3}H	1.87	3.96	6.33	9.06	12.3	16.3	21.4	24.6	28.6	40.4 a
^{14}C	866	1.83	2.93	4.20	5.7	7.53	9.90	11.4	13.2	18.9 ka
^{32}P	2.17	4.60	7.36	10.5	14.3	18.9	24.8	28.6	33.2	47.5 d
^{42}K	1.88	3.99	6.38	9.14	12.4	16.4	21.5	24.8	28.8	41.2 h
^{51}Cr	4.23	8.95	14.3	20.5	27.8	36.7	48.3	55.6	64.6	92.4 d
^{59}Fe	6.84	14.5	23.2	33.2	45.0	59.5	78.2	90.0	104	150 d
^{60}Co	800	1.69	2.71	3.88	5.26	6.95	9.14	10.5	12.2	17.5 a
^{131}I	1.23	2.60	4.15	5.95	8.07	10.7	14.0	16.1	18.7	26.8 d
^{137}Cs	4.56	9.66	15.4	22.1	30.0	39.7	52.1	60.0	69.7	99.7 a
^{182}Ta	17.5	37.0	59.2	84.7	115	152	200	230	267	382 d
^{192}Ir	11.3	23.9	38.2	54.8	74.3	98.2	129	149	173	247 d
^{198}Au	410	869	1.39	1.99	2.70	3.57	4.69	5.40	6.27	8.97 d
^{226}Ra	243	515	823	1.18	1.60	2.12	2.78	3.20	3.72	5.32 ka

For half-lives of additional radionuclides see page 150
Die Halbwertzeiten weiterer Radionuklide siehe Seite 150
Pour les périodes des autres radionucléides, voir page 150
Periodo de vida media de otros radionúclidos, vease página 150

The residual activity of a radionuclide after a given time can be found in table 6.4.2. next page. For example I 131 after 18 days, it amounts to 21.3 % of the initial activity.

Die von einem Radionuklid nach einer bestimmten Zeit noch vorhandene Restaktivität läßt sich aus der Tabelle 6.4.2 herauslesen. Sie beträgt z.B. für J 131 nach 18 Tagen noch 21,3 % der Anfangsaktivität.

L'activité résiduelle d'un radionucléide peut être obtenue à partir de la table 6.4.2. Pour l'Iode 131, par ex. l'activité résiduelle après 18 jours est 21,3 % de l'activité initiale.

La actividad residual de un radionúclido que permanece después de un tiempo determinado se puede leer en la tabla 6.4.2. P. ej. para el I 131 después de 18 días, importa el 21,3 % de la actividad inicial.

6.4.2 Residual activity after different time intervals
Restaktivität nach verschieden langen Zeiten
Activité résiduelle après différents temps
Actividad residual después de diferentes periodos de tiempo

Residual activity in % of the initial activity − Restaktivität in % der Anfangsaktivität − Activité résiduelle en % de l'activité initiale − Actividad residual en % de la actividad inicial — Time − Zeit − Temps − Tiempo

Nuclide — Nuklid Nuclide — Núclido $T_{1/2}$					Time — Zeit — Temps — Tiempo					%
	0.5	1	2	3	4	5	6	7	8	9
	10	12	14	16	18	20	22	24	26	28
	30	35	40	45	50	55	60	65	70	75
	80	90	100	110	120	130	140	150	160	170
	200	230	260	290	320	350	380	410	440	470
^{3}H 12.3 a	97.2	94.5	89.3	84.4	79.8	75.4	71.3	67.4	63.7	60.2	a
	56.9	50.9	45.4	40.6	36.3	32.4	28.9	25.9	23.1	20.6	
^{14}C 5.7 ka	94.1	88.6	78.4	69.4	61.5	54.4	48.2	42.7	37.8	33.5	ka
	29.6	23.2	18.2	14.3	11.2	8.79	6.89	5.40	4.24	3.32	
^{32}P 14.3 d	97.6	95.3	90.8	86.5	82.4	78.5	74.8	71.2	67.9	64.7	d
	61.6	55.9	50.7	46.1	41.8	37.9	34.4	31.2	28.4	25.7	
	23.4	18.3	14.4	11.3	8.86	6.95	5.46	4.28	3.36	2.64	
^{42}K 12.4 h	97.2	94.6	89.4	84.6	80.0	75.6	71.5	67.6	63.9	60.5	h
	57.2	51.1	45.7	40.9	36.6	32.7	29.2	26.1	23.4	20.9	
	18.7	14.1	10.7	8.08	6.11	4.62	3.49	2.64	2.0	1.51	
^{51}Cr 27.8 d	98.8	97.5	95.1	92.8	90.5	88.3	86.1	84.0	81.9	79.9	d
	77.9	74.1	70.5	67.1	63.8	60.7	57.8	55.0	52.3	49.8	
	47.3	41.8	36.9	32.6	28.7	25.4	22.4	19.8	17.5	15.4	
^{59}Fe 45 d	99.2	98.5	97.0	95.5	94.0	92.6	91.2	89.8	88.4	87.1	d
	85.7	83.1	80.6	78.2	75.8	73.5	71.3	69.1	67.0	65.0	
	63.0	58.3	54.0	50.0	46.9	42.9	39.7	36.7	34.0	31.5	
	29.2	25.0	21.4	18.4	15.7	13.5	11.6	9.92	8.50	7.29	
^{60}Co 5.26 a	99.5	98.9	97.8	96.8	95.7	94.7	93.6	92.6	91.6	90.6	Mo *)
	89.6	87.7	85.7	83.9	82.1	80.3	78.5	76.8	75.2	73.5	
	71.9	68.1	64.5	61.0	57.7	54.7	51.7	49.0	46.4	43.9	
	41.5	37.2	33.3	29.9	26.8	24.0	21.5	19.3	17.3	15.5	
^{131}I 8.07 d	95.8	91.8	84.2	77.3	70.9	65.1	59.7	54.8	50.3	46.2	d
	42.4	35.7	30.0	25.3	21.3	18.0	15.1	12.7	10.7	9.03	
^{137}Cs 30 a	98.9	97.7	95.5	93.3	91.2	89.1	87.1	85.1	83.1	81.2	a
	79.4	75.8	72.4	69.1	66.0	63.0	60.2	57.4	54.8	52.4	
^{182}Ta 115 d	94.2	93.0	91.9	90.8	89.7	88.6	87.6	86.5	85.5	84.5	d
	83.5	81.0	78.6	76.2	74.0	71.8	69.7	67.6	65.6	63.6	
	61.7	58.1	54.7	51.5	48.5	45.7	43.0	40.5	38.1	35.9	
	30.0	25.0	20.9	17.4	14.5	12.1	10.1	8.45	7.05	5.88	
^{192}Ir 74.3 d	99.5	99.1	98.2	97.2	96.3	95.4	94.6	93.7	92.8	92.0	d
	91.1	89.4	87.8	86.1	84.5	83.0	81.5	79.9	78.5	77.0	
	75.6	72.1	68.9	65.7	62.7	59.9	57.1	54.5	52.1	49.7	
	47.4	43.2	39.3	35.8	32.6	29.7	27.1	24.7	22.5	20.5	
^{198}Au 2.7 d	99.5	98.9	97.9	96.8	95.8	94.8	93.8	92.8	91.8	90.8	h
	89.9	88.0	86.1	84.3	82.5	80.7	79.0	77.4	75.7	74.1	h
	88.0	77.4	59.8	46.3	35.8	27.7	21.4	16.6	12.8	9.92	d

*) Months − Monate − Mois − Meses

162

6.5   Dosage of radium sources
        Dosierung von Radiumpräparaten
        Détermination de la dose des sources de radium
        Dosificación de fuentes de radio

6.5.1   Exposure rate of point sources
        Dosisleistung punktförmiger Präparate
        Débit d'exposition des sources ponctuelles
        Rendimiento de fuentes puntiformes

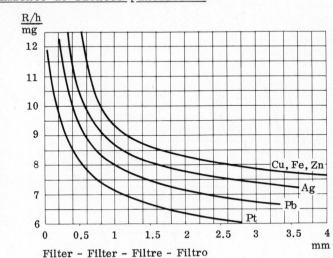

Filter - Filter - Filtre - Filtro

Filter Filter Filtre Filtro	Exposure rate at a distance of 1 cm from the source Dosisleistung in 1 cm Entfernung vom Präparat Débit d'exposition à 1 cm de distance de la source Indice d'exposición a 1 cm de distancia de la fuente			R/h mg
	Filtration - Filterung - Filtration - Filtración			
mm	Pt	Pb	Ag	Cu,Fe,Zn
0.1	10.8	–	–	–
0.2	9.6	–	–	–
0.3	8.8	11.0	–	–
0.4	8.5	10.0	11.5	–
0.5	8.15	9.4	10.5	(13.0)
0.6	7.8	8.9	9.9	11.5
0.8	7.4	8.3	9.1	10.0
1.0	7.15	8.0	8.7	9.3
1.5	6.7	7.5	8.1	8.6
2.0	6.3	7.15	7.8	8.3
2.5	6.1	6.9	7.6	8.1
3.0	–	6.7	7.4	7.8
3.5	–	–	7.2	7.7
4.0	–	–	–	7.6

Lit.: 1. GLASSER, O. et al.: Physical Foundations of Radiol.,
         2. Edit., New York: Harper & Row 1952
      2. MITCHELL, R.G.: Brit.J.Radiol. 29, 631 (1956)
      3. MINDER, W.: Dosimetrie rad. Stoffe, Wien: Springer 1961

6.5.2 Dosage of linear sources
       Dosierung von linearen Präparaten
       Doses pour des sources linéaires
       Dosificación de fuentes lineales

0.5 mm Pt Filtration - Filterung - Filtration - Filtración

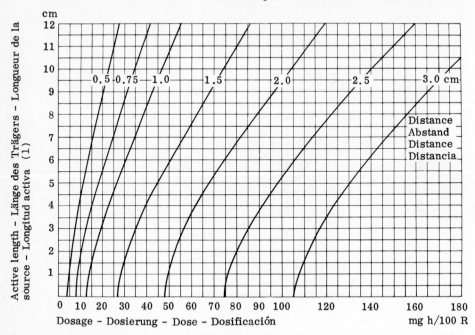

Active length - Länge des Trägers - Longueur de la source - Longitud activa (1)

Dosage - Dosierung - Dose - Dosificación   mg h/100 R

1	mg h required to give a dose of 100 R Zum Erreichen einer Dosis von 100 R erforderliche mg h mg h nécessaires pour obtenir une dose de 100 R mg h necesarios para alcanzar una dosis de 100 R						$\frac{mg\ h}{100\ R}$
	Distance from source - Abstand vom Träger - Distance de la source - Distancia de la fuente						cm
cm	0.5	0.75	1.0	1.5	2.0	2.5	3.0
0.5	3.8	8.3	13	27	49	75	106
1	4.5	8.5	14	28	50	76	108
2	5.8	10	16	31	52	80	112
3	7.5	12	19	35	57	85	117
4	9.0	15	23	39	62	92	123
5	11	18	26	45	68	98	131
6	12	21	31	50	75	106	139
8	18	28	39	63	90	122	157
10	23	35	47	74	105	141	175
12	28	42	55	87	120	160	-

Lit.: 1. PATERSON, R., PARKER, H.M.: Brit.J.Radiol.11,252,313 (1938)
      2. QUIMBY, E.H.: Radiology 43, 572 (1944)
      3. MEREDITH, W.J.: Radium Dosage, Edinburgh: Livingstone 1947
      4. YOUNG, M.E.J., BATHO, H.F.: Brit.J.Radiol. 37, 38 (1964)
      5. IAEA Atlas of Radiation Dose Distributions, IV, Vienna 1972

6.5.3 Dosage of planar sources
Dosierung von flächigen Präparaten
Doses pour des applicateurs plans
Dosificación de fuentes planos

0.5 mm Pt Filtration - Filterung - Filtration - Filtración

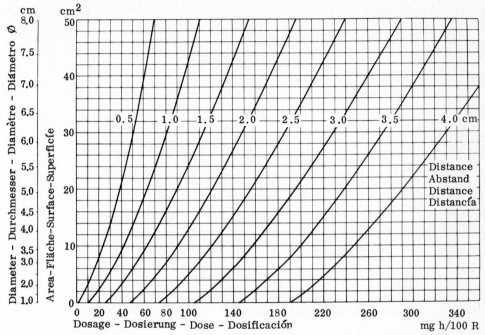

Diameter - Durchmesser - Diamètre - Diámetro ∅

Area - Fläche - Surface - Superficie

Dosage - Dosierung - Dose - Dosificación   mg h/100 R

| Distance |
| Abstand |
| Distance |
| Distancia |

mg h required to give a dose of 100 R
Zum Erreichen einer Dosis von 100 R erforderliche mg h $\frac{\text{mg h}}{100\ R}$
mg h nécessaires pour obtenir une dose de 100 R
mg h necesarios para alcanzar una dosis de 100 R

∅	Area Fläche Surface Superficie	Distance from source Abstand vom Träger Distance de la source Distancia de la fuente							cm
cm	cm^2	0.5	1.0	1.5	2.0	2.5	3.0	3.5	4.0
1.6	2.0	7.2	18	35	58	85	119	159	204
2.3	4.0	12	25	43	67	96	130	170	217
2.8	6.0	16	32	50	75	105	140	181	228
3.2	8.0	20	36	56	83	113	150	190	238
3.6	10	23	42	63	90	121	158	200	247
4.4	15	31	53	77	107	139	177	220	270
5.0	20	38	63	90	122	156	196	239	292
5.7	25	45	73	102	135	172	213	257	312
6.2	30	51	81	114	148	187	230	274	331
6.7	35	56	89	124	161	200	246	291	350
7.1	40	61	96	135	173	214	261	307	(367)
7.6	45	64	104	145	185	227	276	323	–
8.0	50	70	111	154	196	240	290	336	–

Lit.: See pages - Siehe Seiten - Voir pages - Ver páginas 163/164

6.5.4　Evaluation of the minimum dose in interstitial therapy
Ermittlung der Minimaldosis bei Spickung
Evaluation de la dose minimale pour les applications inter-
stitielles
Evaluación de la dosis minima en el applicación intersticial

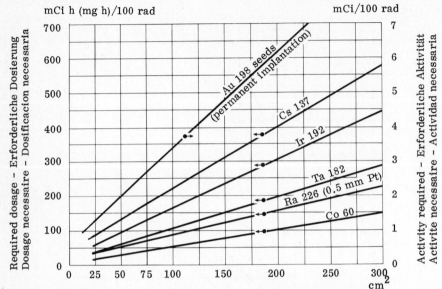

mCi h (mg h)/100 rad

Required dosage - Erforderliche Dosierung
Dosage necessaire - Dosificacion necessaria

mCi/100 rad

Activity required - Erforderliche Aktivität
Activite necessaire - Actividad necessaria

Surface of the target volume - Oberfläche des Zielvolumens
Surface du volume cible - Superficie de la volumen blanco

mg h (mCi h) required to obtain 100 rad in the target volume Zum Erreichen von 100 rad im Zielvolumen erforderliche mg h (mCi h) mg h (mCi h) nécéssaires pour obtenir 100 rad dans le volume-cible mg h (mCi h) necessarios para obtener 100 rad dentro del volumen blanco							
Nuclide Nuklid Nucléide Nuclido	Surface area of the target volume - Ober- fläche des Zielvolumens - Surface du volume cible - Superficie de la volumen blanco cm^2						
	25	50	100	150	200	250	300
Radium 226; 0.5 mm Pt 　　　　(mg h/100 rad)	35	56	87	122	156	192	225
Co 60 (mCi h/100 rad)	16	28	52	74	102	125	150
Ta 182　　　"	38	61	105	151	195	240	280
Ir 192　　　"	62	95	165	235	305	375	445
Cs 137　　　"	90	133	220	310	406	490	570
Au 198 (mCi/100 rad)	1.30	2.00	3.35	4.75	6.20	7.60	8.90

Lit.: 1. LAUGHLIN, J.S., et al.: Am.J.Roentgenol. 89, 470 (1963)
      2. GOODWIN, P.N., QUIMBY, E.M., MORGAN, R.H.: Physical Founda-
         tions of Radiology, New York, London: Harper and Row 1970
      3. BUSCH, M.: Strahlenther., Sonderband 64 (1967)
      4. DIN 6809/2, Berlin: Beuth-Verlag 1975
See also - Siehe auch - Voir aussi - Ver tambien 163 - 164

6.6 I 131 activity required for irradiation of the thyroid gland with a specified dose

Erforderliche J 131 Aktivität zur Bestrahlung der Schilddrüse mit einer bestimmten Dosis

Activité d'I 131 nécessaire pour obtenir une dose donnée dans la thyroide

Actividad necesaria del I 131 para obtener una dosis deseada en la glándula tiroidea

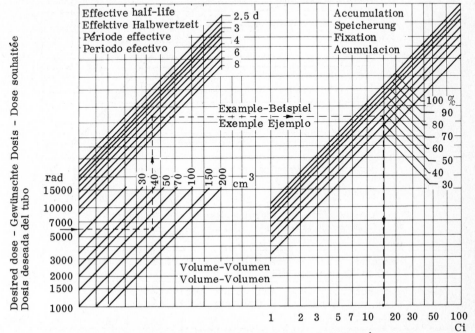

Activity required - Erforderliche Aktivität - Activite nécessaire - Actividad necesaria

Effective half-life and the accumulation must be determined in n each individual case by the iodine uptake test before administration of the therapeutic dose. The dotted line shows an example.

Die effektive Halbwertzeit und die Speicherung müssen in jedem Einzelfall vor der Verabreichung der therapeutischen Dosis durch den Jodtest bestimmt werden. Die gestrichelte Linie zeigt ein Beispiel.

La période effective et la fixation doivent êtra déterminées pour chaque cas particulier grâce aux tests à I 131 avant l'administration de la dose thérapeutique.

El valor del tiempo promedio efectivo y la acumulación se establecerán en cada caso individualmente antes de la administración de la dosis terapeútica por la prueba de compresión. La línea punteada muestra un ejemplo.

Lit.: 1. JOYET, G., MILLER, N.: Ann.Radiol. 5, 21 (1962)

6.7 Exposure rate during handling of Tc 99m and I 131 sources
Dosisleistung beim Umgang mit Tc 99m und J 131
Débit d'exposition à distance de sources de Tc 99m et de I 131
Exposición en trato con fuentes de Tc 99m y I 131

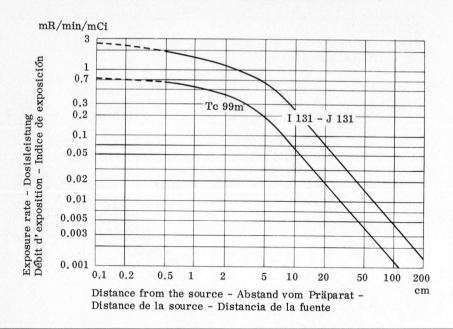

Distance from the source - Abstand vom Präparat -
Distance de la source - Distancia de la fuente

Distance Abstand Distance Distancia	Exposure rate - Dosisleistung - Débit d'exposition - Indice de exposición mR/min							
	For activity of - Bei einer Aktivität - Pour une activité - Con una actividad mCi							
cm	1	2	5	10	20	50	100	150
Tc 99m 0.1	(0.75)	(1.5)	(3.75)	(7.5)	(15)	(38)	(75)	(113)
0.2	(0.70)	(1.4)	(3.5)	(7.0)	(14)	(35)	(70)	(105)
0.5	0.65	1.3	3.25	6.5	13	32.5	65	98
1	0.55	1.1	2.75	5.5	11	27.5	55	83
2	0.42	0.84	2.10	4.2	8.4	21.0	42	63
5	0.19	0.38	0.95	1.9	3.8	9.5	19	29
10	0.052	0.104	0.26	0.52	1.04	2.6	5.2	7.8
20	0.019	0.038	0.095	0.19	0.38	0.95	1.9	2.9
50	0.004	0.008	0.020	0.040	0.08	0.20	0.40	0.60
100	0.0013	0.0026	0.007	0.013	0.26	0.07	0.13	0.20
150	0.0008	0.0016	0.004	0.008	0.016	0.04	0.08	0.12
I 131 - J 131 0.1	(2.5)	(5.0)	(12.5)	(25)	(50)	(125)	(250)	(375)
0.2	(2.3)	(4.6)	(11.5)	(23)	(46)	(115)	(230)	(345)
0.5	1.9	3.8	9.5	19	38	95	190	285
1	1.6	3.2	8.0	16	32	80	160	240
2	1.2	2.4	6.0	12	24	60	120	180
5	0.65	1.3	3.2	6.5	13	32	65	98
10	0.25	0.5	1.25	2.5	5	12.5	25	38
20	0.075	0.15	0.37	0.75	1.5	3.7	7.5	11.2
50	0.015	0.03	0.075	0.15	0.3	0.75	1.5	2.25
100	0.0045	0.009	0.022	0.045	0.09	0.22	0.45	0.68
150	0.0027	0.0054	0.0135	0.027	0.054	0.135	0.27	0.40

6.8   Exposure rate in the vicinity of patients treated with I 131
      Dosisleistung in der Umgebung von J 131-Patienten
      Débit d'exposition au voisinage des malades traités par I 131
      Exposición en la vecindad de pacientes tratados con I 131

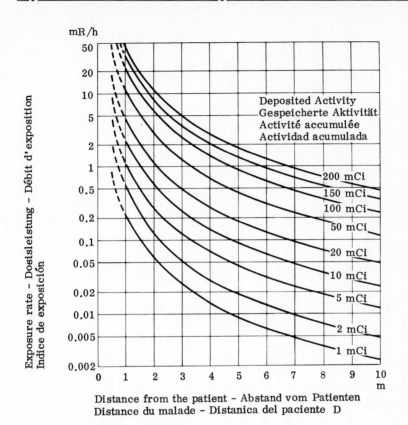

Distance from the patient - Abstand vom Patienten
Distance du malade - Distanica del paciente D

Distance Abstand Distance Distancia D m	Exposure rate - Dosisleistung - Débit d'exposition - Indice de exposición mR/h								
	When activity of ^{131}I deposited in the thyroid gland is - Bei einer in der Schilddrüse gespeicherten ^{131}J Aktivität von - Pour une activité d' ^{131}I fixée dans la thyroide de - Por una actividad de ^{131}I acumulada en la glandula tiroides de: mCi								
	1	2	5	10	20	50	100	150	200
0.5	(0.9)	(1.8)	(4.5)	(9.0)	(18)	(45)	(90)	(140)	(180)
1	0.23	0.46	1.15	2.3	4.6	11.5	23	35	46
1.5	0.10	0.20	0.50	1.0	2.0	5.0	10	15	20
2	0.06	0.12	0.29	0.58	1.2	2.9	5.8	8.6	11.5
3	0.026	0.05	0.13	0.26	0.51	1.28	2.56	3.8	5.1
4	0.014	0.028	0.072	0.14	0.29	0.72	1.44	2.16	2.88
5	0.009	0.018	0.046	0.092	0.18	0.46	0.92	1.38	1.84
6	0.006	0.012	0.032	0.064	0.13	0.32	0.64	0.96	1.28
7	0.005	0.010	0.024	0.047	0.094	0.24	0.47	0.70	0.94
8	0.004	0.007	0.018	0.036	0.072	0.18	0.36	0.54	0.72
10	0.002	0.005	0.012	0.023	0.046	0.12	0.23	0.35	0.46

6.9 Dose to critical organs in different scanning procedures - Strahlenbelastung der kritischen Organe bei verschiedenen szintigraphischen Untersuchungen - Doses aux organes critiques pour différents examens scintigraphiques - Dosis en órganos críticos en diferentes examenes scintigraficos

Organ Organ Organe Organo	1.	2.	3.	$T_{1/2}$	Chemical form Verbindung Forme chimique Especie quimica	Activity Aktivität Activité Actividad µCi	Critical organs Kritische Organe Organes critiques Organos críticos	Dose Dosis Dose Dosis rad
Brain Hirn Cerveau Cerebro	^{131}I ^{131}J	β^-,γ	1-24 h	8.0 h	Serum albumin	350-500	Blood-Blut-Sang-Sangre Thyreoidea Whole body-Ganzkörper-Corps entier-Todo el cuerpo	2.5-3.5 7-25 0.7-1
	^{203}Hg	β^-,γ	2-24 h	47 d	Neohydrin	750	Kidneys-Nieren-Reins-Rinones	315
	^{197}Hg	K,γ	2-4 h	27 d	Neohydrin	750	"	32
					$HgCl_2$	750	"	48
	^{99m}Tc	γ	30 min	6.0 h	Pertechnetat	5000-10000	Intestine-Darm-Intestin-Intestino	1
Heart Herz Coeur Corazón	^{131}I ^{131}J	β^-,γ	5-10 min	8.0 d	Serum albumin	300-400	Blood-Blut-Sang-Sangre Thyreoidea Whole body-Ganzkörper-Corps entier-Todo el cuerpo	2-2.8 6-20 0.6-0.8
	^{99m}Tc	γ	5 min	6.0 h	Serum albumin	3000-4000	Blood-Blut-Sang-Sangre Whole body-Ganzkörper-Corps entier-Todo el cuerpo	0.5 0.2
	^{113m}In	γ	10 min	5 min	Serum albumin	1000-3000	"	0.015
Liver Leber Foie Higado	^{198}Au	β^-,γ	30 min	2.7 d	Colloidal Au	150-400	Liver-Leber-Foie-Higado Spleen-Milz-Rate-Bazo	6-20 3.5-30
	^{131}I ^{131}J	β^-,γ	10-20 min	8.0 d	Rose bengal	100-300	Liver-Leber-Foie-Higado Thyreoidea	0.1-0.3 5-15
	^{99m}Tc	γ	15-20 min	6.0 h	Colloidal Au	1000-3000	Liver-Leber-Foie-Higado Spleen-Milz-Rate-Bazo	0.3-1.6 0.2-1.3

1. Isotope - Isotope - Isotope - Isótopo 2. Type of decay - Zerfallsart - Type de décroissance - Tipo de desintegración 3. Time between application and examination - Zeit zwischen Verabreichung und Untersuchung - Temps entre l'administration et l'examen - Tiempo entre la administración y examen

Organ	Isotope		Time		Compound	Dose	Target organ	~5 local 20-30
Lungs Lungen Poumons Pulmones	^{131}I ^{131}J	β^-,γ	5 min	8.0 h	Makroagg.HSA	300	Lungs-Lungen-Poumons-Pulmones Thyreoidea	~5 local 20-30
	^{51}Cr	K,γ	0.5-3 h	28 d	Makroagg.HSA	1000	Lungs-Lungen-Poumons-Pulmones	3-5
	^{90m}Tc	γ	0.5-3 h	6.0 h	Makroagg.HSA Colloid	1000-2000		0.6
Lymph nodes Lymphknoten Ganglions Nud.linfát.	^{198}Au	β^-,γ	24 h	2.7 d	Colloidal Au	200	Site of injection Injektionsstelle Point d'injection Lugar de la inyección	200-5000
Spleen Milz Rate Bazo	^{51}Cr	K	30 min	28 d	Erythrocytes	400-1000	Spleen-Milz-Rate-Bazo	12-20
	^{197}Hg	K	1 h	2.7 d	BMPH incub. Blood,Blut	300-500	Kidneys-Nieren-Reins-Rinones	20-23
Kidneys Nieren Reins Rinones	^{203}Hg	β	1 h	47 d	Neotydrin	100-150	"	42-63
					Salyrgan	100-160	"	16-24
	^{197}Hg	K	1 h	2.7 d	Neohydrin	100-200	"	6.3-8.4
					$HgCl_2$	200-300		13-16
	^{99m}Tc	γ	1 h	6.0 h	Tc-Fe Komplex	2000	"	1.2
Thyreoidea	^{131}I	β^-	24-48 h	8.0 d	NaJ	25-100	Thyreoidea	25-50
	^{125}I	K	24-48 h	60 d	NaJ	15-50	Thyreoidea	6-18
	^{99m}Tc	γ	20-30 min	6.0 h	Pertechnetat	500-1000	Thyreoidea Intestine-Darm-Intestin- Intestino	0.1-0.2 0.1-0.2
Bone Knochen Os Huesos	^{85}Sr	K	24 h	65 h	$Sr(NO_3)_2$ $SrCL_2$	50-100	Bone-Knochen-Os-Huesos	2-4
	^{87m}Sr	IT	3-4 h	2.8 h	$Sr(NO_3)_2$	3000	Bone-Knochen-Os-Huesos	0.3
	^{99m}Tc	γ	2-4 h	6.0 h	Polyphosphat	5000-10000	Bladder-Blase-Vessie-Vejiga	1-2
	^{18}F	β^+,EC	1-3 h	1.8 h	Fluorid	2000-3000	Stomach-Magen-Estomac-Estómago Bladder-Blase-Vessie-Vejiga	1-1.5 4-6
Tumor diagnosis	^{67}Ga	K,EC	2-3 d	78 h	Citrat	2000-3000	Bone marrow-Knochenmark Moelle-Médula Liver-Leber-Foie-Hígado	1-2

6.10   Radionuclide generators
        Radionuklid Generatoren
        Générateurs de radionucléide
        Sistemas generadores de radionúclidos

Parent - Mutter - Père - Padre				Daughter - Tochter - Fils - Hijo			
Nuclide Nuklid Nucléide Núclido	*) $T_{1/2}$	**)	γ-Energy γ-Energie γ-Energie γ-Energía keV	Nuclide Nuklid Nucléide Núclido	*) $T_{1/2}$	**)	γ-Energy γ-Energie γ-Energie γ-Energía keV
^{99}Mo	2.8 d	β^-,γ	740 780	^{99m}Tc	6 h	γ	140
^{113}Sm	118 d	EC,γ	255	^{113m}In	1.7 h	γ	393
^{132}Te	3.2 d	β^-,γ	230	^{132}I	2.3 h	β^-,γ	670
^{87}Y	3.3 d	EC,β^+,γ	483	^{87m}Sr	2.8 h	γ	388
^{68}Ge	275 d	EC	–	^{68}Ga	68 min	β^+,γ	511
^{137}Cs	30 a	β^-	–	^{137m}Ba	2.6 min	γ	662
^{81}Rb	4.7 h	EC,β^+,γ	–	^{81m}Kr	13 s	γ	190
^{77}Br	58 h	β^-,γ	240 520	^{77m}Se	18 s	γ	161
^{191}Os	16 d	γ	130	^{191m}Ir	4.9 s	γ	129

*) $T_{1/2}$ = Time in which 1/2 of the radioactive atoms disintegrate
        (radioactive half-life)
        Zeit, in der die Hälfte der radioaktiven Atome zerfallen
        sind
        Temps au bout duquel la moitié des atomes radioactifs
        se sont désintégrés
        Tiempo en el cual la mitad de los átomos radioactivos
        se desintegran

**)   = Type of decay
            Zerfallsart
            Type de désintégration
            Tipo de decaimiento

EC   = Electron capture
            Elektroneneinfang
            Capture électronique
            Captura de electrones

6.11 Some formulas used in counting statistics
Einige Formeln zur Zählstatistik
Quelques formules utilisées en statistiques
Algunas fórmulas para el tratamiento estadístico de datos

Arithmetic mean of a set of data $(x_1 \ldots x_i \ldots x_n)$
Arithmetischer Mittelwert eines Datensatzes $(x_1 \ldots x_i \ldots x_n)$
Moyenne arithmétique d'un ensemble de données $(x_1 \ldots x_i \ldots x_n)$
Media aritmética de un conjunto de valores $(x_1 \ldots x_i \ldots x_n)$

$$\bar{x} = \frac{1}{n} \sum_{i=1}^{n} x_i$$

Standard deviation of a set of data
Standardabweichung eines Datensatzes
Ecart type pour un ensemble de données
Desviación standard de un conjunto de datos

$$s_x^2 = \frac{1}{n-1} \left\{ \sum_{i=1}^{n} x_i^2 - \frac{\left(\sum_{i=1}^{n} x_i \right)^2}{n} \right\} \quad ; \quad s_x = \sqrt{s_x^2}$$

Standard deviation of the mean
Standardabweichung des Mittelwertes
Ecart type de la moyenne
Desviación standard del valor medio

$$s_{\bar{x}} = \frac{s_x}{\sqrt{n}}$$

Covariance of two sets of data $(x_1 \ldots x_i \ldots x_n \ldots)$ and $(x_1 \ldots y_i \ldots y_n)$
Kovarianz zweier Datensätze $(x_1 \ldots x_i \ldots x_n)$ und $(y_1 \ldots y_i \ldots y_n)$
Covariance de deux ensembles de données $(x_1 \ldots x_i \ldots x_n)$ et $(y_1 \ldots y_i \ldots y_n)$
Covariancia de dos series de valores $(x_1 \ldots x_i \ldots x_n)$ y $(y_1 \ldots y_i \ldots y_n)$

$$s_{xy} = \frac{1}{n-1} \sum_{i=1}^{n} (x_i - \bar{x})(y_i - \bar{y}) = \frac{1}{n-1} \left\{ \Sigma x_i y_i - \frac{1}{n} \Sigma x_i \Sigma y_i \right\}$$

Correlation coefficient of two sets of data
Korrelationskoeffizient zweier Datensätze
Coefficient de correlation entre deux ensembles de données
Coeficiente de correlación de dos conjuntos de valores

$$r_{xy} = \frac{s_{xy}}{s_x s_y}$$

Poisson distribution - Poissonverteilung
Distribution de Poisson - Distribución de Poisson

$$P(x) = \frac{\bar{x}^x d^{-\bar{x}}}{x!}$$

Normal distribution - Normalverteilung
Distribution normale - Distribución normal

$$P(x) = \frac{1}{\sqrt{2\pi s_x}} \; e^{-\frac{(x-\bar{x})^2}{2s_x^2}}$$

Standard deviation of a Poisson or normal distribution
Standardabweichung einer Poisson oder Normalverteilung
Ecart type pour une distribution de Poisson ou pour une distribution normale
Desviación standard de una distribución de Poisson o normal

$$s_x = \sqrt{\bar{x}} \approx \sqrt{x}$$

Probability (W) that $\bar{x}$ lies in an interval $x \pm k \cdot s_x$
Wahrscheinlichkeit (W), daß $\bar{x}$ in einem Intervall $x \pm k \cdot s_x$ liegt
Probabilité (W) pour que $\bar{x}$ soit dans l'intervalle $x \pm k \cdot s_x$
Probabilidad (W) de que $\bar{x}$ este en un intervalo $x \pm k \cdot s_x$

k	0.675	1	1.65	2	2.58	3
W (%)	50	68.3	90	95.4	99	99.73

Standard deviation for difference of measured values
Standardabweichung für die Differenz von Meßwerten
Ecart type pour des différences de mesures
Desviación standard de la diferencia de valores experimentales

$$s_f = \sqrt{s_x^2 + x_y^2} \qquad f = x - y$$

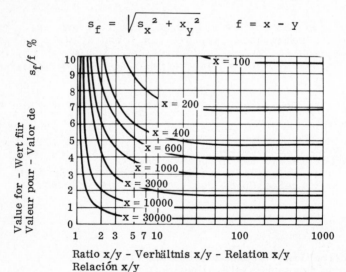

Ratio x/y - Verhältnis x/y - Relation x/y
Relación x/y

Lit.: 1. BURINGTON, R.: Handbook of Mathematical Tables and
          Formulas, New York, St.Louis, San Francisco, Toronto,
          London: Mc Graw-Hill 1965
       2. SACHS, L.: Statistische Auswertungsmethoden, Berlin,
          Heidelberg, New York: Springer Verlag 1969

Table of contents - Inhaltsverzeichnis
Table des matières - Tabla de materias

7.1 Factors affecting patient exposure
Faktoren, die die Patientenexposition beeinflussen
Facteurs intervenant sur l'exposition du malade
Factores que influyen en la exposición de los pacientes

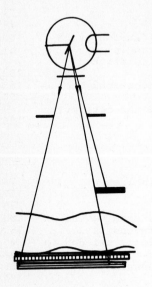

Kilovoltage - Spannung
Tension - Tensión

Tube current - Röhrenstrom
Courant du tube - Corriente del tubo

Filter - Filter - Filtre - Filtro

Collimator - Blende
Diaphragme - Colimador

Focus-film distance - Fokus-Film-Abstand
Distance foyer-film
Distancia foco-película

Shielding - Abdeckung
Écran de protection - Placa de proteción

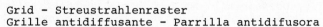

Grid - Streustrahlenraster
Grille antidiffusante - Parrilla antidifusora

Film/intensifying screens
Film/Verstärkerfolien
Film/écrans renforçateurs
Pelicula/cartulinas de refuerzo

Image amplifier-TV - Bildverstärker-FS
Amplificateur de brillance-TV
Intensificador de imagen-TV

Fluoroscopic exposure time - Durchleuchtungs-
zeit - Durée de la radioscopie - Tiempo de la
radioscopia

Number of radiographs - Anzahl der Aufnahmen
Nombre de clichés - Cantidad de radiografias

Development - Entwicklung
Développement - Revelado

Lit.: 1. SEELENTAG, W.: Dtsch.med.Wschr. 86, 2513 (1961)
      2. TER-POGOSSIAN, M.: The physical aspects of diagnosic radio-
         logy, New York, Evanston, London: Hoeber Medical Div. 1967
      3. DUTREIX, J., BISMUTH, V., LAVAL-JEANTET, M.: Traité de
         Radiodiagnostic, Vol. 1, Paris: Masson & Cie. 1969
      4. STIEVE, F.E.: Strahlenschutz in Forschung und Praxis 10,
         148 (1970)

7.2 Recommended kilovoltage ranges for radiography
     Empfehlenswerte Spannungsbereiche für Röntgenaufnahmen
     Domaines de tensions recommandés pour les radiographies
     Márgenes de tensión recomendables para las radiografias

Grid – Streustrahlenraster – grille antidiffusante – parilla antidifusora		kV	
	Without–ohne–sans–sin	25 – 35	Mammography – Mammographie Mammographie – Mamografia
		40 – 50	Soft tissue (leg, neck) Weichteile (Bein, Hals) Parties molles (jambe, cou) Partes blandas (pierna, cuello)
	With – mit – avec – con	60 – 75	Petrous bone, cervical spine, shoulder, thorax, gall bladder, kidneys, knee, lower leg Felsenbein, Halswirbelsäule, Schulter, Thorax, Gallenblase, Nieren, Knie, Unterschenkel Rocher, colonne cervicale, épaule, thorax, vésicule biliaire, reins, genou partie inférieure de la jambe Hueso occipital, raquis cervical, hombro, thorax, vejiga biliar, rinon, rodilla, pierna
		75 – 90	Skull, thoracic and lumbar spine a.p., lung (children), trachea a.p., pelvis, femur Schädel, Brust- und Lendenwirbelsäule a.p., Lunge (Kinder), Trachea a.p., Becken, Oberschenkel Crâne, colonne dorsale et lombaire a.p., poumon (enfants), trachée-artère a.p., bassin, fémur Cráneo, raquis dorsal y lumbar a.p., pulmon (ninos), traquéa a.p., pelvis, femur
		90 – 125	Lung, lumbar spine lat., trachea lat., stomach, small intestine, colon, obstetric radiography Lunge, Lendenwirbelsäule und Trachea seitl., Magen, Dünndarm, Dickdarm, Schwangerschaftsaufnahmen Poumon, colonne lombaire lat., trachée-artère lat., estomac, intestin grêle, colon, radiographie obstétrique Pulmón, raquis lumbar lat., tráques lat., éstomago, intestino delgado, colon, radiografia obstetrica
		125 – 150	Lung lat. – Lunge seitl. Poumon lat. – Pulmón lat.

Lit.: 1. WIDENMANN, L.: Radiography 29, 81 (1963)
      2. ELEGEM van, P.: J. Belge Radiol. 55, 271 (1972)

7.3 Conversion factors for radiography
Umrechnungsfaktoren für Röntgenaufnahmen
Facteurs de conversion pour la radiographie
Factores de conversión para la radiografía

7.3.1 Variation of mAs with tube voltage
mAs-Produkt bei Änderung der Röhrenspannung
Variation du nombre de mAs avec la tension d'alimentation
Producto mAs con el cambio del voltaje del tubo

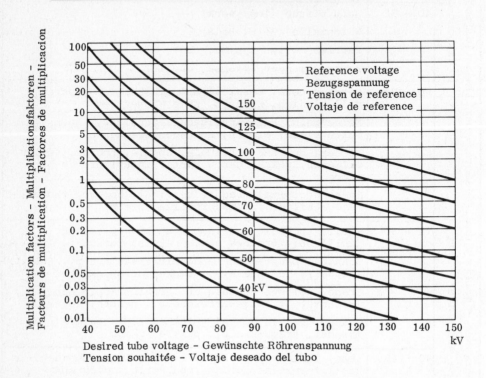

Desired tube voltage - Gewünschte Röhrenspannung
Tension souhaitée - Voltaje deseado del tubo

Reference voltage Bezugs- spannung Tension de réference Voltaje de reference	Multiplication factors - Multiplikationsfaktoren - Facteurs de multiplication - Factores de multiplicación f_{kV}								
	Desired tube voltage - Gewünschte Röhrenspannung - Tension souhaitée - Voltaje deseado del tubo kV								
	40	50	60	70	80	90	100	125	150
40 kV	1	0.3	0.13	0.06	0.03	0.016	0.014	0.0051	0.0021
50 kV	3.05	1	0.40	0.19	0.10	0.05	0.03	0.013	0.0051
60 kV	7.6	2.49	1	0.46	0.24	0.13	0.09	0.037	0.020
70 kV	16.4	5.4	2.2	1	0.53	0.28	0.19	0.077	0.037
80 kV	32	10.5	4.2	1.95	1	0.56	0.37	0.15	0.072
90 kV	57.6	19	7.6	3.51	1.80	1	0.66	0.27	0.13
100 kV	87.5	28.7	11.5	5.34	2.74	1.52	1	0.41	0.20
125 kV	214	70	28	13	6.7	3.7	2.44	1	0.48
150 kV	442	145	58	27	13.8	7.7	5.05	2.07	1

7.3.2 Variation of mAs with changing focus-film-distance (FFD)
mAs-Produkt bei Änderung des Fokus-Film-Abstandes (FFA)
Variation du nombre de mAs avec la distance foyer-film (DFF)
Cambio de la mAs con la distancia foco-película (DFP)

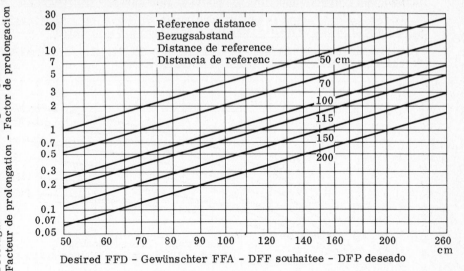

Desired FFD - Gewünschter FFA - DFF souhaitee - DFP deseado

7.3.3 mAs when body thickness differs from a given value d
mAs bei einer gegenüber dem Wert d abweichenden Körperdicke
mAs quand l'épaisseur de corps diffère d'une valeur d donnée
mAs cuando el espesor del cuerpo difiere de un valor d dado

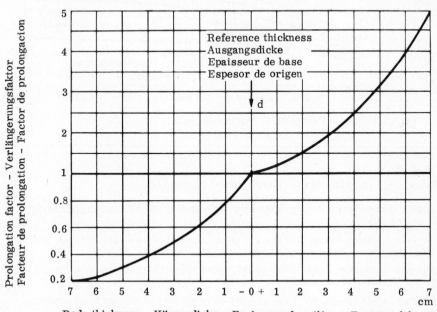

Body thickness - Körperdicke - Epaisseur du milieu - Expesor del cuerpo

7.4 Prolongation factors for exposure time in radiography with the use of antidiffusion grids (grid factors)

Verlängerungsfaktoren für die Belichtungszeit von Röntgenaufnahmen bei Verwendung von Streustrahlenrastern (Rasterfaktoren)

Facteurs pour l'accroissement du temps de pose en radiographie avec des grilles antidiffusantes (facteurs de grille)

Factores de prolongación para el tiempo de exposición usando rejillas antidifusoras (factores de rejilla)

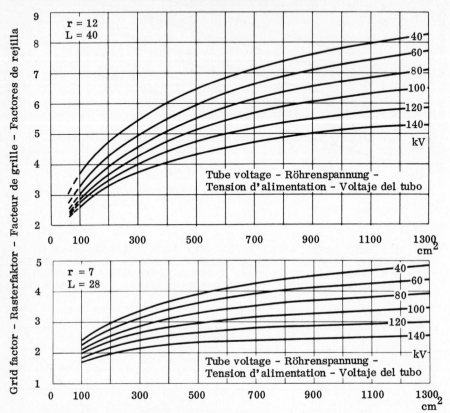

Field size - Feldgröße - Champ - Campo

r = Grid ratio - Schachtverhältnis - Rapport de grille - Razón de rejilla

L = Lines/cm - Linien/cm - Lames/cm - Lineas/cm

The values given in the graphs are valid for a 17 cm thick body (water phantom).

Die aus den graphischen Darstellungen zu entnehmenden Werte gelten für einen Körper (Wasserphantom) von 17 cm Dicke.

Les valeurs données dans les graphiques sont valables pour un corps (eau) de 17 cm d'épaisseur.

Los valores indicados en las gráficas son válidos para un cuerpo (muneco de agua) de un grosor de 17 cm.

7.5 <u>Nomogram for estimating the skin dose in diagnostic radiology</u>
<u>Nomogramm zur Abschätzung der Hautdosis in der Diagnostik</u>
<u>Nomogramme pour l'estimation de la dose à la peau en diagnostic</u>
<u>Nomograma para la estimacion de dosis en la piel en diagnóstico</u>

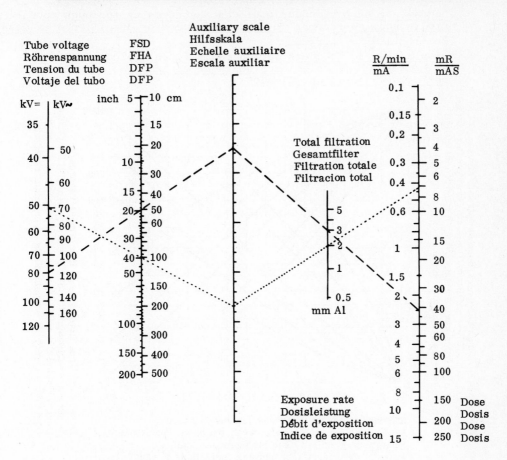

Examples - Beispiele - Exemples - Ejemplos:

(---) Fluoroscopy - Durchleuchtung - Radioscopie - Fluoroscopia
80 kV~; FSD - FHA - DFP - DFP 50 cm; Filter - Filter - Filtre -
Filtro 3 mm Al; Skin dose rate - Hautdosisleistung - Débit de
dose à la peau - Rendimiento de dosis en la piel ≅ 2.5 $\frac{R/min}{mA}$

(...) Radiography - Aufnahme - Radiographie - Radiografía 50 kV=;
FSD - FHA - DFP - DFP 100 cm; Filter - Filter - Filtre - Filtro
2 mm Al; Skin dose - Hautdosis - Dose à la peau - Dosis en la
piel ≅ 40 $\frac{mR}{mAs}$

Lit.: 1. WACHSMANN, F.: Fortschr. Röntgenstr. <u>6</u>, 728 (1951)

7.6 <u>Depth dose curves for typical radiations used in diagnosis,</u>
<u>and ratio of dose at entrance field/film dose (average values)</u>

<u>Dosisabfall der in der Diagnostik verwendeten typischen Strah-</u>
<u>lungen und Verhältnis Dosis-Strahleneintrittsfeld/Filmdosis</u>

<u>Rendements en profondeur pour des rayonnements typiques de ra-</u>
<u>diodiagnostic; rapport de la dose à l'entrée du milieu à la dose</u>
<u>au film (valeurs moyennes)</u>

<u>Disminución de la dosis de las radiaciones típicas usadas en</u>
<u>el diagnóstico, y relaciones dosis en el campo de entrada/dosis</u>
<u>película (valores aproximados)</u>

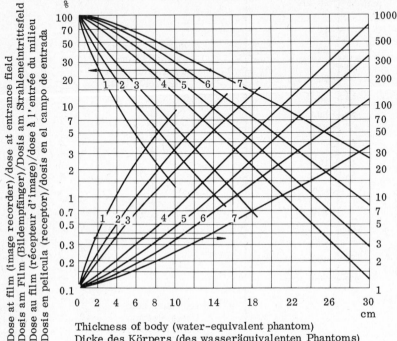

Thickness of body (water-equivalent phantom)
Dicke des Körpers (des wasseräquivalenten Phantoms)
Epaisseur de milieu (fantôme équivalent eau)
Espesor del cuerpo (del fantoma equivalente al agua)

Radiations used - Benützte Strahlungen - Rayonnements utilisés - Radiaciones utilizadas						
Curve Kurve Courbe Curva	Application Anwendung Examen Aplicación	Tube voltage Röhrenspannung Tension du tube Voltaje del tubo kV	FSD FHA DFP DFP cm	Filtration Filterung Filtration Filtración mm	Field Feld Champ Campo cm	HVL HWSD CDA CHR mm
1	Mammography	Mo (17.7 keV)	45	0.1 Mo	15 x 15	∿1 Al
2	Dental X-rays	45 kV∿	15	1.5 Al	5 ∅	1.1 Al
3	Extremities	50 kV∿	50	1.5 Al	20 x 20	1.3 Al
4	General	60 kV∿	120	2 Al	30 x 30	1.6 Al
5	General	80 kV=	120	2 Al	30 x 30	2.4 Al
6	General	120 kV=	120	2 Al	30 x 30	3.4 Al
7	General	150 kV=	120	5 Al	30 x 30	0.3 Cu

7.7 Exposure (D) at the detector and resolution for radiographs
Dosis (D) am Detektor und Auflösung für Röntgenaufnahmen
Exposition (D) sur le détecteur et résolution pour radiographies
Exposición (D) en el detector y resolución para radiografias

Type of radiography - Aufnahmeart - Type de radiographie - Tipo de radiografia		Exposure Dosis (D)	Resolution *)
Non-screen radiography - Folienlose Aufnahme - Radiographie sans écran - Radiografia sin pantalla		10 - 100 mR	10 - 40
Photofluorography-Schirmbildfotographie Radiophotographie-Fluorografía		3 - 5 mR	1.5 - 3
Radiography with screens Aufnahmen mit Folien Radiographie avec écrans Radiografía con pantallas	High definition Feinzeichnend Haute définition Grano fino	0.7 - 2 mR	8 - 12
	Universal-Standard	300 - 800 µR	7 - 9
	High speed Hochverstärkend Rapide - Rápida	200 - 300 µR	5 - 7
	Rare earths Seltene Erden Terres rares Tierras raras	100 - 25 µR	4 - 7
Photographic recording from image intensifier Fotographische Aufzeichnung vom Bildverstärkerschirm Enregistrement photographique dè amplificateur de luminance Registro fotografico de intensificador de imagen		$\dfrac{70 - 100 \text{ mm:}}{50 - 100 \text{ µR}}$ $\dfrac{\text{Cine:}}{2 - 20 \text{ µR}}$	1.5 - 4 1.0 - 3.5
Photographic recording from TV monitor Fotographische Aufzeichnung vom FS-Schirm En registrement photographique de TV moniteur Registro fotografico de TV pantalla		0.5 - 2.0 µR	0.8 - 1.2
Xeroradiography - Xeroradiographie Xeroradiographie - Xeroradiografía		10 - 100 mR	**)

*) Periods/mm - Perioden/mm - Périodes/mm - Periodos/mm
**) Incomparable - Unvergleichbar - Incomparable - Incomparable

Lit.: 1. ROSSMANN, K.: Phys.Med.Biol., 9, 551 (1964)
      2. DUTREIX, J., BISMUTH, V., LAVAL-JEANTET, M.: Traité de radiodiagnostic, Vol. I, Paris: Masson 1969
      3. WIDENMANN, L.: Rö.Praxis 26, 85 (1973)
      4. PUPPE, D.: Grundlagen u. Anwendungsmöglichkeiten, Ergebn. med. Radiologie, Bd. III, Stuttgart: Thieme 1971

7.8 <u>Sensitivity of X-ray films (average values) – Empfindlichkeit von Röntgenfilmen (Richtwerte) –</u>
<u>Sensibilité des films radiographiques (valeurs moyennes) – Sensibilidad de películas para</u>
<u>rayos X (valores aproximados)</u>

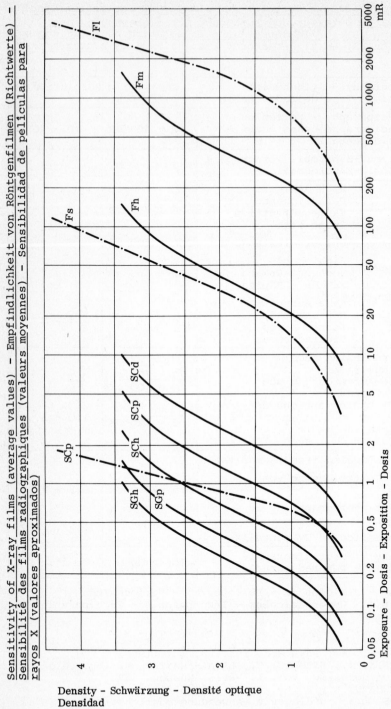

Density - Schwärzung - Densité optique
Densidad

For abbreviations see right page – Abkürzungen siehe rechte Seite – Pour les abréviations voir page de
droite – Para abreviaciones, ver página derecha

Lit.: 1. Brochures – Firmenprospekte – Prospectur des divers fabricants – Prospectos de casas de
comercio
2. BORCKE, E.: Röntgenpraxis 12, 277 (1970)
3. KRAFT, A., NAHRSTEDT, U., WIDENMANN, L.: Röntgenpraxis 28, 264 (1975)
4. Authors' measurements – Eigene Messungen – Mesures personelles – Medidas propias

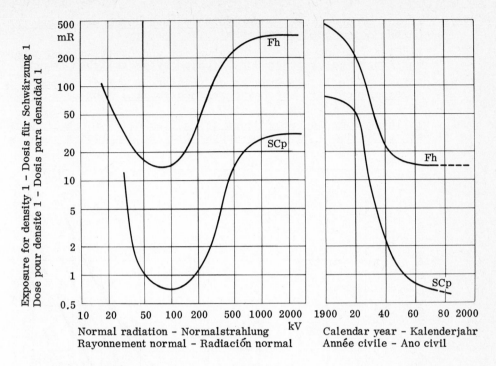

Normal radiation - Normalstrahlung kV
Rayonnement normal - Radiación normal

Calendar year - Kalenderjahr
Année civile - Ano civil

Intensifying screens - Verstärkerfolien - Ecrans renforçateurs - - Pantallas reforzadoras:

S = Screen/film-combination - Film/Folien-Kombination - Combinaison film/écran - Combinación-pantalla/película

F = Non screen films - Folienlose Filme - Films sans écrans - Películas sin pantalla

C = Ca WO_4

G = $Gd_2 O_2$ S: Tb

h = High-speed - Hochverstärkend - Rapides - Amplificación elevada

p = Parspeed - Universal - Standard - Universal

d = High definition - Feinzeichnend - Haute définition - Resolución fina

X-ray films - Röntgenfilme - Films radiologiques - Películas radiologicas

s = High sensitivity-Hochempfindlich-Grande sensibilité-Alta sensibilidad (diagnostic, industrial, personal monitoring)

l = Low sensitivity-Wenig empfindlich-Faible sensibilité-Baja sensibilidad (industrial, personnel monitoring)

m = Mamography - Mammographie - Mammographie - Mamografía

Processing - Entwicklung - Développement - Relevado

—— = Automatic processing - Maschinenentwicklung - Développement automatique - Procesado automático

-·- = Manual processing - Handentwicklung - Développement manuel - Relevado manual

7.9　Effect of developer temperature (t) and developing time (T) on the doses needed for equal film density

Einfluß von Entwicklertemperatur (t) und -zeit (T) auf die zur Erzielung gleicher Schwärzungen erforderlichen Dosen

Influence de la température du révélateur (t) et du temps de développement (T) sur les doses nécessaires pour obtenir un noircissement donné

Influencia de la temperatura (t) y tiempo (T) de revelado sobre las dosis necesarias para alcanzar densidades iguales

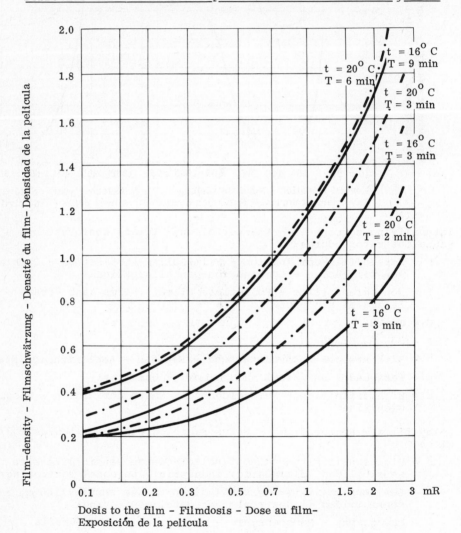

Film–density – Filmschwärzung – Densité du film – Densidad de la pelicula

Dosis to the film – Filmdosis – Dose au film–
Exposición de la pelicula

Lit.: 1. STIEVE, F.E.: Strahlenschutz in Forschung und Praxis, 7, 71, Freiburg: Rombach-Verlag 1967

Table of contents - Inhaltsverzeichnis
Table des matières - Tabla de materias

Type Bezeichnung Désignation Nombre	Frequency or energy Frequenz bzw. Energie Fréquence ou énergie Frecuencia o energía	Wavelength Wellenlänge Longueur d'onde Longitud de onda
Electromagnetic waves of low frequency - Elektromagnetische Oscillations électromagnétiques de basse fréquence -		
Short waves Kurzwellen Ondes courtes Ondas cortas	27.1 Mc/s - MHz [2]) 433.92 " " 2450 " "	11.06 m 69.14 cm 12.24 cm
Infrared Infrarot Infrarouge Rayos infrarrojos	0.2-1.5 eV	5-0.7 µm
Visible light Sichtbares Licht Lumière visible Luz visible	1.5-3 eV	760-400 nm
Ultraviolet Ultraviolett Ultra-violet Radiación ultravioleta	3-12 eV	400-230 nm
X-Rays - Röntgenstrahlen -		
Very soft X-rays Sehr weiche Strahlen Rayons X tres mous Rayos X may blandos	< 6-12 keV	> 6 nm
Low energy X-rays Weiche Strahlen Rayons X mous Rayos blandos	20-60 keV	6-2 nm
Medium-energy X-rays Mittelharte Strahlen Rayons X semi-durs Rayos semiduros	60-150 keV	2-0.8 nm
Orthovoltage X-rays Harte Strahlen Rayons durs (classiques) Rayos duros	150-400 keV	0.8-0.3 nm
High voltage X rays Sehr harte u. γ-Strahlen Rayons extra durs et γ Rayos muy duros y γ	400-3000 keV	0.3-0.04 nm

HVD [1]) GHWT PDA PHR H_2O	Applications Anwendungen Applicâtions Aplicaciones	Mechanism of action Wirkungsmechanismus Mécanisme d'action Mecanismo de acción
	Schwingungen niederer Frequenz - Oscilaciónes electromagnéticas de frecuencia baja
0.5-1 cm 2-9 cm 0.5-2 cm	Heat therapy Wärmetherapie Thermothérapie Termoterapia	Increase in blood circulation Durchblutungssteigerung Amélioration de la circulation sanguine Aumento de la circulación
1 mm	Light therapy Lichttherapie Photothérapie Fototerapia	Superficial heating Oberflächige Erwärmung Augmentation superficielle de la température Calentamiento superficial
0.5 mm	Light therapy Lichttherapie Photothérapie Fototerapia	Heat and photochemical effects Wärme und photochemische Wirkungen Chaleur et action photochimique Calor y efectos fotoquimicos
	Ultraviolet therapy Ultraviolett-Therapie Thérapie par UV Fototerapia con UV	Photochemical effects Photochemische Wirkungen Action photochimique Efectos fotoquímicos
	Rayons X - Rayos X
0.2 mm	Skin therapy [4]) Hauttherapie Radiothérapie des lésions cutanées Terapia dermatologica	Cell damage by ionization Zellschädigungen durch Ionisation Lésions cellulaires par ionisation Lesión tisular por ionización LET [3]) 6-3 keV/µm ID [3])150-100/µm
2-30 mm	Skin and subcutaneous therapy [5]) Haut- u.Unterhautther. Radiothérapie cutanée et souscutanée Terapia cutánea y subcutánea	" LET ∿ 2.6 keV/µm ID ∿ 70/µm
30-70 mm	Intermediate therapy [5]) Halbtiefentherapie Thérapie semi- profonde Terapia semiprofunda	" LET 2.5-1.5 keV/µm ID 90-50/µm
7-8 cm	Deep therapy [6]) Tiefentherapie Radiothérapie profonde Terapia profunda	" LET 1.5-0.5 keV/µm ID ∿ 50-15/µm
8-12 cm	" " [7])	" LET 0.5-0.25 keV/µm ID ∿ 15-8/µm

Type Bezeichnung Désignation Nombre	Frequency or energy Frequenz bzw. Energie Fréquence ou énergie Frecuencia o energîa	Wavelength Wellenlänge Longueur d'onde Longitud de onda
Megavoltage rays [8]) Ultraharte Strahlen Rayons X de très haute énergie Rayos X ultraduros	3-50 MeV	< 0.04 nm
Corpuscular radiations - Korpuskularstrahlen -		
Alpha rays Alphastrahlen Rayons alpha Rayos alfa	1-10 MeV	-
Beta rays Betastrahlen Rayons beta Rayos beta	1-3 MeV	-
Fast electrons [9]) Schnelle Elektronen Electrons accélérés Electrones rápidos	5-50 MeV	-
Neutrons [10]) Neutronen Neutrons Neutrones	0.02 eV - 60 MeV	-
Protons [11]) Protonen Protons Protones	50-200 MeV	-

Definitons - Definitionen - Définitions - Definiciónes

[1]) HVD = Half-value depth (tissue)
   GHWT = Gewebe-Halbwerttiefe
   PDA = Profondeur demi atténuation tissulaire
   PHR = Profundidad hemi reductora en tejido

[2]) Mc/s = M cycle/s   = Megahertz/s
        = 10^6 Schwingungen/s
        = M oscillations/s
        = M oscilaciónes/s

HVD [1]) GHWT PDA PHR H_2O	Applications Anwendung Applications Aplicaciones	Mechanism of action Wirkungsmechanismus Mécanisme d'action Mecanismo de acción
$\sim$ 15 cm	Deep therapy Tiefentherapie Thérapie des lésions profondes Terapía profunda	Cell damage Zellschädigung Lésion cellulaire Lesión tisular LET $\sim$ 0.25 keV/μm ID $\sim$ 7/μm

Rayonnements corpusculaires - Radiación corpuscular

5 μm	Contact therapy Kontaktbestrahlung Thérapie de contact Terapía de contacto	" LET keV/μm ID μm^{-1} $\sim$ 150-30 $\sim$ 5000-1000
5 mm	Skin therapy Hauttherapie Thérapie cutanée Terapía dermatológica	" $\sim$ 0.3-0.2 $\sim$ 10-6
2-10 cm	Intermediate therapy Halbtiefentherapie Thérapie semiprofonde Terapía semiprofunda	" LET $\sim$ 0.2 keV/μm ID $\sim$ 7/μm
2-15 cm	In experimental stage Im Versuchsstadium Stade expérimental Fase experimental	" LET 1.5 keV/μm ID $\sim$ 50/μm
5-20 cm	"	" LET 0.3-0.15 ID $\sim$ 10-5/ m

[3]) LET - ID   See page - Siehe Seite - Voir page - Ver pagina 37-39

[4]) See page - Siehe Seite - Voir page - Ver pagina 87, 100 - 103
[5]) "   "   "   "   87 - 103
[6]) "   "   "   "   104 - 111
[7]) "   "   "   "   118 - 127
[8]) "   "   "   "   126 - 129
[9]) "   "   "   "   132 - 133
[10]) "   "   "   "   134
[11]) "   "   "   "   135

8.2 Data for the "reference man" (adult) – Angaben über den "Referenz-Menschen" (Erwachsener) – Données sur "l'homme référence" (adulte) – Datos sobre el "hombre-referencia" (adulto)

8.2.1 Organ weights – Organgewichte – Poids des organes – Peso del órgano

	Male / Mann / Homme / Hombre (g)	Female / Frau / Femme / Mujer (g)	Average value / Mittelwert / Valeur moyenne / Valor medio (g)
Total body – Ganzkörper – Corps entier – Cuerpo total	70000	58000	
Skeletal muscles – Skelettmuskulatur – Muscles du squelette – Esqueleto muscularios	28000	17000	
Skeleton (with bone marrow etc.) – Skelett (mit Knochenmark usw.) – Squelette (y compris la moelle etc.) – Esqueleto (incluida médula, etc.)	10000	6800	
Skin – Haut – Peau – Piel	2600	1790	
Subcutaneus tissue – Unterhautgewebe – Tissus souscutanés – Tejido subcutáneo	7500	13000	
Fat – Fett – Graisse – Grasa	16000	13500	
Red bone marrow – Rotes Knochenmark – Moelle rouge – Médula roja	1500	1300	
Yellow bone marrow – Weißes Knochenmark – Moelle jaune – Médula blanca	1500	1300	
Blood – Blut – Sang – Sangre	5500	4100	4800
Gastrointestinal tract (without contents) – Magen-Darm-Kanal (ohne Inhalt) – Tractus gastrointestinal (sans contenu) – Tubo digestivo (vacío)	1200	1200	
Gastrointestinal tract (content) – Magen-Darm-Kanal (Inhalt) – Tractus gastrointestinal (contenu) – Tubo digestivo (contenido)	1000	1000	
Liver – Leber – Foie – Hígado	1800	1400	1600
Brain – Hirn – Cerveau – Cerebro	1400	1200	1300
Lungs – Lungen – Poumons – Pulmones	1150	880	
Lymphoid tissue – Lymphatisches Gewebe – Tissu lymphoide – Tejido linfático	700	580	
Heart – Herz – Coeur – Corazón	330	240	
Kidneys – Nieren – Reins – Rinones	310	275	
Spleen – Milz – Rate – Bazo	180	150	
Pancreas – Bauchspeicheldrüse – Pancréas – Páncreas	100	85	
Salivary glands – Speicheldrüsen – Glandes salivaires – Glándulas salivales	85	70	
Thyroid gland – Schilddrüse – Thyroïde – Tiroides	20	17	
Thymus – Thymus – Thymus – Timo			
Testicles – Hoden – Testicules – Testículos	35	–	10
Prostate gland – Prostata – Prostate – Prostata	16	–	

8.2.2 Daily food intake – Tägliche Nahrungsaufnahme – Quantités ingérées quotidiennement – Dieta alimenticia diaria

	Male Mann Homme Hombre	Female Frau Femme Mujer	Child 10 a Kind 10 a Enfant 10 a Niño 10 a
		g/24 h	
Water balance – Wasserhaushalt – Bilan en eau – Balance de agua			
Ingestion – Aufnahme – Ingestion – Ingestión			
In fluids – In Getränken – Dans les boissons – En bebidas	1950	1400	1400
In food – In der Nahrung – Dans l'alimentation – En comidas	700	450	400
By oxidation – Durch Verbrennung – Par oxydation – Por oxidación	350	250	200
Total – Zusammen – Total – Total	3000	2100	2000
Excretion – Ausscheidung – Sécrétion – Secreción			
Urine – Urin – Urine – Orina	1400	1000	1000
Feces – Stuhl – Fèces – Deposiciones	100	90	70
Insensible loss – Unmerkbar – Perte inapparente – Pérdidas imperceptibles	850	600	580
Sweat – Schweiß – Sueur – Transpiración	650	420	350
Total – Zusammen – Total – Total	3000	2100	2000

8.2.3 Breathed air – Atemluft – Air inhalé – Aire inhalado

	Male Mann Homme Hombre	Female Frau Femme Mujer	Child 10 a Kind 10 a Enfant 10 a Niño 10 a
		ℓ/8 h	
Light activity – Leichte Arbeit – Travail facile – Actividad moderada	9600	9100	6240
Nonoccupational activity – Freizeit – Activité non professionnelle – Tiempo libre	9600	9100	6240
Resting – Schlaf – Sommeil – Durante el sueño	3600	2900	2300
Total – Zusammen – Total – Total: Liters–Liter–Litres–Litros/24 h	22800	~21000	~15000

Lit.: 1. ICRP Publ. 23, Oxford: Pergamon Press (1975)

8.3   <u>Dose/effect relationships of ionising radiations</u>
<u>Dosis/Wirkung Beziehungen ionisierender Strahlungen</u>
<u>Relations dose/effet pour les rayonnements ionisants</u>
<u>Relación dosis/efecto de radiaciones ionizantes</u>

8.3.1   <u>Target theory (based on mathematical considerations)</u>
<u>Treffertheorie (auf mathematischen Überlegungen basierend)</u>
<u>Théorie de la cible (basée sur des considérations mathe-</u>
<u>matiques)</u>
<u>Teoría del blanco (basada en consideraciones matemáticas)</u>

The term "hit" refers to an elementary physical event (e.g., formation of an ion pair) within a "sensitive volume" (e.g., cell nucleus
or chromosome). Single hits (n = 1), plotted logarithmically, give
linear dose-effect curves; curves for multiple hits (n = 2...n) are
sigmoidal.

"Treffer" nennt man ein physikalisches Elementarereignis (z.B. Aus-
lösung eines Ionenpaares) innerhalb eines "empfindlichen Volumens"
(z.B. Zellkern oder Chromosom). Eintreffervorgänge (n = 1) ergeben
logarithmisch dargestellt geradlinige Mehrtreffervorgänge (n = 2...n)
sigmatoide Dosiswirkungskurven.

Le terme "coup" se rapporte à un évènement physique élémentaire (par
exemple: formation d'une paire d'ions) à l'intérieur d'un volume
sensible (par exemple: noyau cellulaire ou chromosome). Le modèle à
un coup (n = 1) représenté avec des ordonnées logarithmiques, conduit
à une courbe dose-effet linéaire; les modèles à plusieurs coups (n =
2...n) conduisent à des sigmoides.

El término "pegar en el blanco" o "impacto" se refiere a un evento
físico elemental (por ejemplo formación de pares de iones) en un
"volumen sensible" (por ejemplo núcleos celulares o cromosomas).
Procesos de impacto unitarios (n = 1) ofrecen perfiles lineales en
representaciones logarítmicas de las relaciones de dosis/efecto,
mientras que para procesos de impacto múltiple (n = 2...n) son sigmoi-
dales.

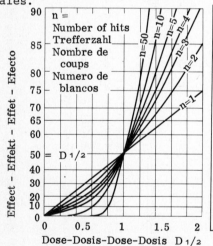

Object	Effect	n
Drosophila	Mutation	1
Viruses - Viren	Inactivation	1
B.coli, prodi-giosus, etc.	Killing-Ab-tötung-Mort Muerta	1
Yeast - Hefe - Levures-Levadura	Damage-Schä-digung-Dom-mage-Daño	3-5
Seeds-Keimlinge-Germes-Semillas	"	5-28
" depending on age " je nach Alter	"	
" and-und-et-y kV	"	1-18
Mammalian cells	"	15-20

Effect - Effekt - Effet - Efecto

Dose-Dosis-Dose-Dosis $D_{1/2}$

Lit.: 1. TIMOFEEFF-RESSOWSKY, N.W., ZIMMER, K.G.: Das Trefferprinzip
     in der Biologie, Leipzig: Hirzel 1947
    2. KELLERER, A.M.: Handbuch der Radiologie, Bd. II/3, Berlin,
     Heidelberg, New York: Springer 1972

8.3.2 Survival rate in cell cultures
Überlebensrate in Zellkulturen
Taux de survie de cultures de cellules
Relación de supervivencia en cultivos celulares

Note - Bemerkungen - Remarque - Nota

D_0 = Dose which reduces the number of surviving cells to the fraction
1/e;

n = "extrapolation number", i.e., the number of survivors, determined by continuation of the linear portion of the damage curve
to its intersection with the ordinate.

D_0 = Dosis, durch die die Zahl der jeweils überlebenden Zellen auf
den 1/e-ten Teil vermindert wird;

n = "Extrapolationsnummer", d.h. die Zahl der Überlebenden, gefunden
durch Verlängerung des geradlinigen Teils der Schädigungskurve
bis zum Schnittpunkt mit der Ordinate.

D_0 = Dose qui réduit le nombre de cellules survivantes à une fraction
1/e;

n = "nombre d'extrapolation", c'est à dire le nombre de survivants
déterminé par extrapolation de la partie linéaire de la courbe
de survie jusqu'à son intersection avec l'axe des ordonnées.

D_0 = Dosis mediante la cual el número de células que sobreviven disminuye a la porción 1/e;

n = "número de extrapolación", es decir el número de sobrevivientes,
que se obtiene prolongando la parte recta de la curva de dañados
hasta que corta el eje de ordenadas.

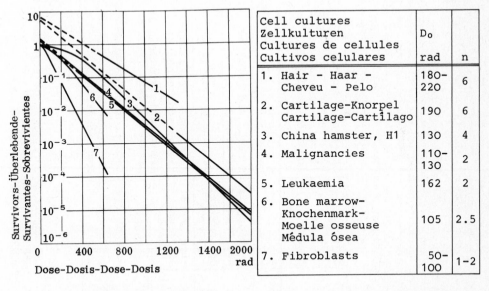

Cell cultures Zellkulturen Cultures de cellules Cultivos celulares	D_0 rad	n
1. Hair - Haar - Cheveu - Pelo	180-220	6
2. Cartilage-Knorpel Cartilage-Cartílago	190	6
3. China hamster, H1	130	4
4. Malignancies	110-130	2
5. Leukaemia	162	2
6. Bone marrow- Knochenmark- Moelle osseuse Médula ósea	105	2.5
7. Fibroblasts	50-100	1-2

Survivors-Überlebende-Survivantes-Sobrevivientes

Dose-Dosis-Dose-Dosis

Lit.: 1.-3. PUCK, T.T., MARCUS, P.I. et al.: J.Exp.Med. 103, 273,
485 (1956) and 106, 485 (1957)
4. TROTT, K.R.: Hdb. der Radiologie, Bd. II/3, Berlin,
Heidelberg, New York: Springer 1972

8.4.1 Relative biological effectivness (RBE) - Relative biologische Wirksamkeit (RBW) - Efficacité biologique relative (EBR) - Efectividad biológica relativa (EBR)

Since the RBE is strongly dependent on the object and its condition, the reaction under consideration, the temporal dose distribution, and extraneous circumstances, only examples can be given here. - Da die RBW stark von dem Objekt und seinem Zustand, der betrachteten Reaktion, der zeitlichen Dosisverabreichung und Nebenumständen abhängig ist, können hier nur Beispiele gegeben werden. - Etant donnée la dépendance marquée de l'EBR suivant le matériel et ses conditions, suivant le test biologique considéré, suivant la distribution de la dose dans le temps et suivant les conditions extérieures, seuls quelques exemples sont présentés. - Dado que la EBR depende en gran medida del objeto y su estado, reacción considerada, suministro de dosis temporal y circunstancias accesorias, solamente se pueden indicar aquí ejemplos.

Group / Gruppe / Groupe / Grupo	Object / Objekt / Matériel / Objeto	Observed reaction / Beobachtete Reaktion / Réaction observé / Reacción observada	LET - LEÜ - TEL - TEL - RBE - RBW - EBR - EBR keV/μm; 0.2 0.5 1 2 5 10 20 50 100 200 500 1000; Ionisation density - Ionisationsdichte / Densité d'ionisation - Densidad de ionización; 6 15 30 60 150 300 600 1500 3000 6000 15000 30000 Pairs/μm
Primitive plants / Pilze	Fungi / Pilze	Mutations 2) Deletions	Reference radiation 1; 2 — 5.5; 5.5 / 74
Higher plants	Arabidopsis, zea, nigella	Somatic and germline mutations 2)	1; 9 16 18; 51-49 22-66 29-89; 11.5 →1.5
Insects	Drosophila, silk worm	Various mutations 2)	1; 1-2 2-4; 1-2.5 4
Mammals / Säugetiere / Mammifère / Mamíferos	Mice, rats / Different tissues	Mutations, transloca-tions, and lethal 2)	1; 1.1-1.2 2 3-6 6
	Fast-growing tissues	Haemopoetic syndrome 1) Damage - death 1)	1; 1.2 1.5 2; 1-3 2-4 5 6
	Lens of eye	Induction of cataracta 3)	1; (2-) 8 (-20)
	Different cells	"Biologic effect" of fractionation 3)	1; single dose 1-1.1; 5 fractions/5 days 0.9-1.7

Lit.: 1. ICRP Report No. 14, Oxford: Pergamon-Press 1969
      2. ICRP Report No. 18, Oxford: Pergamon-Press 1972
      3. BROERSE, J.J.: Europ.J.Cancer. 10, 225 (1974)

8.4.2　Erythema dose as a function of radiation energy
　　　　Erythemdosis bei Strahlungen verschiedener Energie
　　　　Doses d'érythème en fonction de l'énergie du rayonnement
　　　　Dosis eritematosa en función de la energía de la radiación

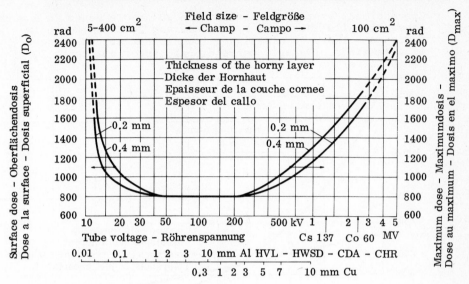

Lit.: 1. REISNER, A.: Fortschr. Röntgenstr. 45, 293 (1932)
　　　 2. TRUMP, J.G.: Radiology 50, 645 (1948)
　　　 3. WACHSMANN, F.: Proceedings of the Congressus Int.Dermatolo-
　　　　　 giae 1967, Vol. 2, Springer: Heidelberg 1968

Note - Bemerkung - Remarque - Nota:

The absorption of soft X-rays in the horny layer of the skin and its steep dose decay respectively the significant build-up above 250 kV makes it possible to irradiate skin with higher surface doses (D_O) at low energies and with higher maximum doses (D_{max}) at high energies, without exceeding the erythema or tolerance threshold.

Die Schwächung in der Hornhaut und der steile Dosisabfall weicher Röntgenstrahlen bzw. der über 250 kV Bedeutung erlangende Aufbaueffekt bewirken, daß bei weichen Strahlungen höhere Oberflächendosen und bei sehr bis ultraharten Strahlungen höhere Maximumdosen (D_{max}) verabreicht werden können als im Bereich von 50 - 200 kV ohne die Erythem- oder Toleranzschwelle zu überschreiten.

L'absorption des rayons X mous dans la couche cornée de la peau et la décroissance rapide de la dose d'une part et d'autre part l'accroissement initial significatif de la dose au dessus de 250 kV permettent d'irradier la peau avec des doses à la surface (D_O) plus élevées pour les rayonnements de basse energie au pour les hautes énergies sans dépasser de seuil érythème où tolerance.

La atenuación en el callo y el escarpado descenso de la dosis de los rayos blandos o sea el efecto de build-up encima de 250 kV da lugar a que se puedan aplicar con rayos blandos dosis superficiales (D_O) y con rayos de alta energía dosis medidas en el máximo (D_{max}) más elevadas como en el intervalo 50 - 250 kV sin sobrepasar el límite erimatoso o de tolerancia.

Lit.: 1. REISNER, A.: Fortschr. Röntgenstr. 45, 293 (1932)
　　　 2. TRUMP, J.G.: Radiology 50, 645 (1948)
　　　 3. WACHSMANN, F.: Proceedings of the Congressus Int.Dermatolo-
　　　　　 giae 1967, Vol. 2, Springer: Heidelberg 1968

8.5.1 <u>Dependence of skin tolerance on field size</u>
<u>Abhängigkeit der Hauttoleranz von der Feldgröße</u>
<u>Variation de la tolérance cutanée avec la taille du champ</u>
<u>Dependencia de la tolerancia de la piel con el campo</u>

Conventional therapy; fractionation 20 single doses in 4 weeks
Konventionelle Therapie; Fraktionierung 20 Einzeldosen in
4 Wochen - Thérapie classique; fractionnement: 20 séances
en 4 semaines - Terapia convencional; fraccionamiento 20
dosis unitarias en 4 semanas

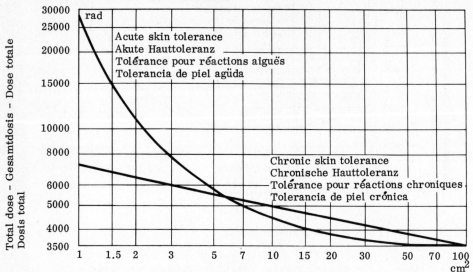

Field size - Feldgröße - Champ - Campo

Field size Feldgröße Champ Campo cm^2	Skin tolerance - Hauttoleranz - Tolérance cutanée - Tolerancia de la piel rad	
	Acute - Akut Aiguë - Aguda	Chronic - Chronisch Chronique - Crónica
1	28 000 rad	7 300 rad
1.5	15 000	6 800
2	11 000	6 400
3	7 800	6 000
5	5 800	5 600
7	5 000	5 300
10	4 500	5 000
15	4 000	4 800
20	3 800	4 500
30	3 700	4 200
50	3 550	3 850
70	3 500	3 700
100	3 500	3 500

Lit.: 1. JOYET, G., HOHL, K.: Fortschr. Rö.Strl. <u>82</u>, 387 (1955)
      2. von ESSEN, C.F.: in Frontiers of Radiation Therapy and
         Oncology, Vol. 6, Basel: S. Karger 1972

8.5.2 Skin reactions as a function of different fractionnation
Hautreaktionen bei verschiedener Fraktionierung
Réactions de la peau pour différents fractionnements
Reacciones de la piel según el fraccionamiento

Conventional therapy - Konventionelle Therapie - Thérapie
classique — Terapía convencional (∿ 200 kV)

100 cm^2 Field size - Feldgröße - Champ - Campo

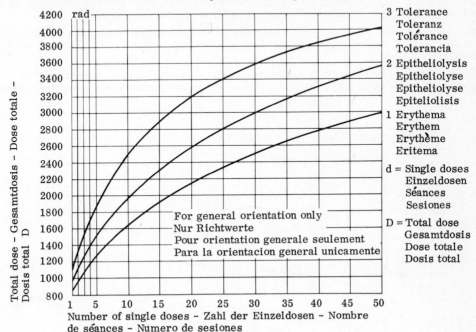

3 Tolerance
Toleranz
Tolérance
Tolerancia

2 Epitheliolysis
Epitheliolyse
Epitheliolyse
Epiteliolisis

1 Erythema
Erythem
Erythème
Eritema

d = Single doses
Einzeldosen
Séances
Sesiones

D = Total dose
Gesamtdosis
Dose totale
Dosis total

For general orientation only
Nur Richtwerte
Pour orientation generale seulement
Para la orientacion general unicamente

Total dose - Gesamtdosis - Dose totale -
Dosis total D

Number of single doses - Zahl der Einzeldosen - Nombre
de séances - Numero de sesiones

Number of single doses Zahl der Einzeldosen Nombre de séances Número de sesiones	Doses for various skin reactions - Dosen zur Erzeugung verschiedener Hautreaktionen - Expositions différentes pour reactions cutanées - Dosis para varias reacciones cutáneas rad					
	1		2		3	
	d	D	d	D	d	D
1	850	850	950	950	1100	1100
2	1000	425	1100	475	1350	550
3	1100	333	1300	366	1600	450
5	1300	260	1550	310	1900	380
7	1500	215	1750	250	2150	308
10	1650	165	1950	195	2500	250
15	1900	125	2300	153	2900	193
20	2150	110	2600	130	3200	160
25	2350	95	2800	112	3400	137
30	2500	85	3000	100	3600	120
35	2650	75	3150	90	3750	107
40	2800	70	3300	83	3850	97
45	2900	65	3450	77	3950	88
50	3000	60	3550	71	4000	80

Lit.: 1. WACHSMANN, F.: Strahlenther. 73, 636 (1943)
2. STRANDQVIST, M.: Acta Radiol. Suppl. LV (1944)

8.6 "Nominal single doses" (NSD) in the fractionated radiotherapy
"Nominale Einzel-Dosen" (NED) bei Fraktionierung
Doses équivalentes en radiothérapie fractionnée (NSD)
Dosis equivalente en la radioterapia fraccionada (NSD) 1-2)

Reference value 1000 rad; proportional transformation in other NSD is possible. In certain tissues deviations may be occur.

Bezugswert 1000 rad; proportionale Umrechnung auf andere NED ist zulässig. Bei gewissen Geweben sind Abweichungen möglich.

NSD équivalent de 1000 rad; une règle de proportionnalité est acceptable pour d'autres NSD. Pour certains tissus des écarts sont possibles.

Valor de referencia 1000 rad; se puede realizar la conversión proporcional a otras NSD. Para ciertos tejidos son posibles desviaciones.

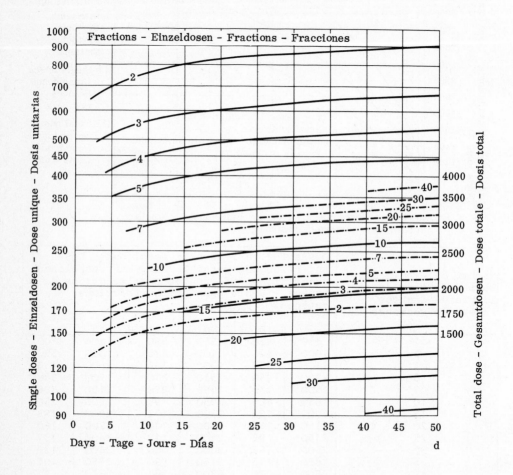

Lit.: 1. ELLIS, F.: Clin.Radiol. 20, 1 (1969)
      2. ELLIS, F. et al.: Brit.J.Radiol. 42, 715 (1969)
      3. KROENING, P.M. et al.: Am.J.Roentgenol. CXII, 803 (1971)

Equivalent single dose - Äquivalente Einzeldosen - Dose équivalente par séance - Dosis únitarias equivalentes										rad
Number of fractions - Zahl der Einzeldosen - Nombre de séances - Número de sesiones										
d*)	2	3	4	5	7	10	15	20	25	30	40
2	635	-	-	-	-	-	-	-	-	-	-
3	670	490	-	-	-	-	-	-	-	-	-
4	690	505	405	-	-	-	-	-	-	-	-
5	705	520	415	350	-	-	-	-	-	-	-
7	720	535	430	365	280	-	-	-	-	-	-
10	760	560	450	380	295	225	-	-	-	-	-
15	795	585	470	395	310	235	172	-	-	-	-
20	825	600	485	410	315	240	177	143	-	-	-
25	840	620	500	420	325	250	182	146	123	-	-
30	860	630	510	430	330	255	186	150	126	110	-
40	890	650	520	445	340	260	192	154	130	113	91
50	910	665	535	455	350	270	196	158	133	115	93

Equivalent total doses - Äquivalente Gesamtdosen - Doses totales équivalentes - Dosis total equivalente

d*)	2	3	4	5	7	10	15	20	25	30	40
2	1170	-	-	-	-	-	-	-	-	-	-
3	1340	1470	-	-	-	-	-	-	-	-	-
4	1580	1515	1620	-	-	-	-	-	-	-	-
5	1410	1560	1660	1750	-	-	-	-	-	-	-
7	1440	1605	1720	1825	1960	-	-	-	-	-	-
10	1520	1680	1800	1900	2065	2250	-	-	-	-	-
15	1590	1755	1880	1975	2170	2350	2580	-	-	-	-
20	1650	1800	1940	2050	2205	2400	2660	2860	-	-	-
25	1680	1860	2000	2100	2275	2500	2760	2920	3075	-	-
30	1720	1890	2040	2310	2550	2790	3000	3150	3300	-	-
40	1780	1950	2080	2225	2380	2600	2980	3080	3250	3390	3640
50	1820	1995	2140	2275	2450	2700	2940	3160	3325	3450	3720

Treatment time Behandlungszeit Durée du traitement Duración del tratamiento Weeks-Wochen Semaines-Semanas	Equivalent doses with 1 - 5 irradiations/week Äquivalente Dosen bei 1 - 5 Bestrahlungen/Woche Dose équivalente à 1 - 5 irradiations/semaine Dosis equivalentes con 1-5 irradiaciones/semana rad									
	Single doses-Einzeldosen Dose unique-Dosis únitarias rad					Weekly dose-Wochendosis Dose hebdomadaire Dosis semanales rad				
	1	2	3	4	5	1	2	3	4	5
1	1000	730	535	430	360	1000	1460	1615	1720	1800
2	780	465	345	280	235	780	930	1030	1120	1175
3	605	360	262	212	178	605	720	790	850	890
4	505	295	220	175	148	505	590	660	700	740
5	435	258	188	152	128	435	515	565	610	645
6	385	230	168	135	114	385	460	505	540	570
7	350	186	152	122	103	350	372	455	490	515

*) d = Duration of the treatment (days) - Behandlungsdauer (Tage) - Durée du traitement (jours) - Duración del tratamiento (dias)

(ret = $rad_{therapy}$)

8.7 Effect of dose protraction on various biological tissues and reactions (average values)

Einfluß der Protrahierung auf verschiedene Gewebe und Reaktionen (Richtwerte)

Influence de l'étalement de la dose sur différents tissus et différentes réactions biologiques (pour orientation seulement)

Efecto de la protracción de la dosis sobre diversos tejidos y reacciones biológicas (para orientación unicamente)

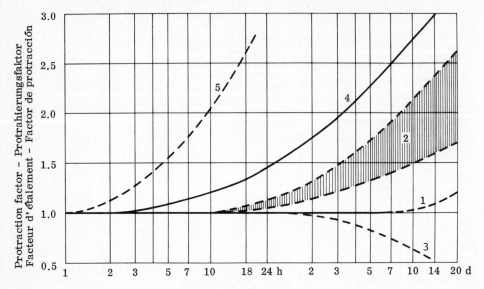

Irradiation time - Bestrahlungsdauer - Durée de l'irradiation
Duración de la radiación

1. Resting cells and mutations - Ruhende Zellen und Mutationen - Cellules au repos et mutations - Células en reposo y mutaciones

2. Tumour cells, killing - Tumorzellen, abtöten - Cellules tumorales, amortir - Destrucción de células tumorales

3. Germ cells - Samenepithel - Cellules germinales - Células seminales

4. Skin erythema - Hauterythem - Erythème cutané - Eritema cutáneo

5. Fast growing tissues - Schnell wachsende Gewebe - Tissus en croissance rapide - Tejidos de crecimiento rápido

Lit.: 1. QUIMBY, E.H., Mc COMB, W.S.: Radiology 29, 305 (1937)
      2. CHAOUL, H., WACHSMANN, F., ROSENBERGER, H.: Strahlenther. 76, 224 (1944)
      3. PATERSON, R.: Treatment of malignant disease by radium and X-rays, Baltimore: Williams and Wilkins 1948

| Time / Zeit / Durée / Tiempo | Protraction factors - Protrahierungsfaktoren[*] / Facteurs d'étalement - Factores de protracción | | | | | f_{ep} [**] |
	f_p1	f_p2	f_p3	f_p4	f_p5	1:2
1 h	1	1	1	1	1	1
2 h	1	1	1	1	1	1
3 h	1	1	1	1.02	1	>1
5 h	1	1	1	1.08	1	1.08
7 h	1	1	1	1.15	≫1	1.12
10 h	1	>1	1	1.20	≫1	1.20
15 h	1	>1	1	1.24	≫1	1.25
18 h	1	>1	1	1.33	≫1	1.30
24 h=1d	1	(1.05-1.1)	1	1.45	≫1	1.35
2 d	1	(1.1 -1.3)	1	1.75	≫1	1.55
3 d	1	(1.2 -1.45)	(>1)	1.95	≫1	1.65
4 d	1	(1.25-1.6)	(>1)	2.15	≫1	1.75
5 d	1	(1.35-1.7)	(>1)	2.25	≫1	1.75
7 d	1	(1.4 -1.9)	(>1)	2.5	≫1	1.8
10 d	(>1)	(1.5 -2.1)	(>1)	2.75	≫1	1.9
14 d	(>1)	(1.6 -2.4)	(>1)	3.05	≫1	2.0
20 d	(>1)	(1.7 -2.6)	(>1)	-	≫1	2.0

[*] "Protraction factor " f_p = protracted dose/short-term dose, both of which produce the same biological effects; (1 - 5 see left page).

"Protrahierungsfaktor" f_p = Dosis protrahiert/Dosis kurzzeitig, bei beiden Verabreichungsarten gleiche biologische Wirkungen; (1 - 5 siehe linke Seite).

"Facteur d'étalement" f_p = dose avec irradiation étalée/dose avec irradiation aiguë qui produisent le même effet biologique; (1 - 5 voir page de gauche).

"Factor de protracción" f_p = dosis protraida/dosis aplicada en breve tiempo obteniéndose con ambas formas de tratamiento los mismos efectos biológicos (1 - 5 ver página izquierda).

[**] "Therapeutic ratio" of dose protraction (e.g., tumor/skin: $f_{ep} = f_{p4}/f_{p2}$). The therapeutic ratio indicates how much the tumor dose can be increased while the reaction to healthy tissue (skin) remains unchanged.

"Elektivitätsfaktor" der Protrahierung (z.B. Tumor/Haut: $f_{ep} = f_{p4}/f_{p2}$). Der Elektivitätsfaktor gibt an, eine um wievielmal höhere Dosis dem Tumor bei gleichbleibender Belastung (Reaktion) des gesunden Gewebes (Haut) gegeben werden kann.

"Facteur de sélectivité" lié à l'étalement (par ex. tumeur/peau: $f_{ep} = f_{p4}/f_{p2}$). Il indique le facteur par lequel la dose à la tumeur peut être multipliée, pour que la réaction des tissus sains reste la même.

"Factor de electividad" de la protracción (p. ej. tumor/piel: $f_{ep} = f_{p4}/f_{p2}$). El factor de electividad indica en que proporción se puede suministrar al tumor una dosis superior, permaneciendo igual el daño (reacción) del tejido (piel) sano.

8.8 Growth of malignant tumours (average values)
Wachstum bösartiger Geschwülste (Richtwerte)
Croissance des tumeurs malignes (valeurs moyennes)
Crecimiento de tumores malignos (valores promedios)

8.8.1 Theory of constant tumour doubling time (t_D)
Theorie der gleichbleibenden Tumor-Verdopplungszeit (t_D)
Théorie du temps de doublement constant de la tumeur (t_D)
Teoría del tiempo constante de duplicación de los tumores (t_D)

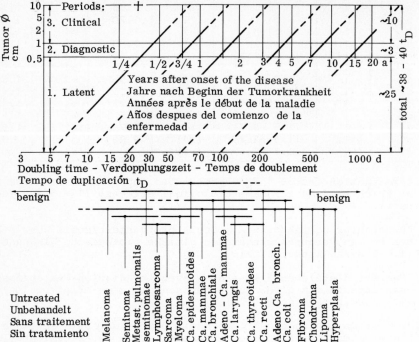

The graph indicates the approximate duration of the latent period, the period of the possible diagnosis and the duration of the clinical phase. In practice many tumours grow faster in the initial phase and more slowly at the end of the clinical phase, than corresponds to the doubling time.

Die Darstellung zeigt die ungefähre Dauer der Entstehungsphase, den frühestmöglichen Zeitpunkt der Diagnose und die Dauer der klinischen Phase. In der Praxis wachsen Tumoren anfangs oft schneller und am Ende der klinischen Phase langsamer als der Verdopplungszeit entspricht.

Le graphique indique la durée approximative de la periode de latence, le moment où le diagnostic est possible et la durée de la phase clinique. En pratique de nombreuses tumeurs grossissent plus vite dans la phase initiale et plus lentement à la fin de la phase clinique que ne le montre le temps de doublement.

La gráfica indica la duración aproximada de la fase de generación, el término de la diagnosis y la duración de la fase clínica. En realidad los tumores crecen al comienzo más rapidamente y al final de la fase clinica más lentamente de lo correspondiente al tiempo de duplicación.

Lit.: 1. COLLINS, V.P. et al.: Am.J.Roentgenol. 76, 988 (1956)
      2. CHARBIT, A. et al.: Europ.J.Cancer. 7, 307 (1971)
      3. OESER, H.: Krebsbekämpfung..., Stuttgart: Thieme 1974

<u>Prognosis for malignant tumours following radiation therapy</u>
         <u>Prognose maligner Tumoren nach Strahlentherapie</u>
         <u>Prognose pour les tumeurs malignes après radiothérapie</u>
         Pronóstico de tumores malignos según la radioterapia

The average values given refer to patients who were treated
between 1945 and 1965 - Die angegebenen groben Richtwerte
beziehen sich auf Patienten, die etwa 1945 - 1965 behandelt
wurden - Valeurs approchées se rapportant à des malades
traites entre 1945 et 1965 - La cifras aproximadas se re-
fieren a pacientes tratados entre 1945 y 1965

Tumour / Tumor / Tumeur / Tumor	Frequency / Häufigkeit / Fréquence / Frecuencia %	5-year survivors / 5-Jahre Überlebende / Survivants à 5 ans / 5 anos supervivencia / Stage-Stadium-Stade-Fase					Remarks / Bemerkungen / Observations / Observaciones
		1	2	3	4	total	
Bronchus	10					5	Inopérable
Collum uteri	9	60	60	30	7	55	Conventional
		75	75	45	10	70	Super voltage therapy
Mamma	8	80	40	-20-		50	Operable
		40	20	-10-		25	Inoperable
Rectum	4.3	40	40	-10-		30	(Intracavitary therapy 80 %)
Corpus uteri	3.4					55	Operable
		55	19			22	Inoperable
Ovarium	3.1	90	60	45	15		
Vulva	0.6	80	60	20	5	30	
Vagina	0.4	60	35	20	9	45	
Vesica urin.	1.7	65	30	15	8	30	
Oesophagus	1.0					3	
M. Hodgkin	0.9	55	40	14		30	(1972∿70 %)
Larynx	0.8	85	70	40	15	65	
Cutis	3	95	90	80		90	
Melanoma	0.7	70	30	12	∿0	60	
Lingua	0.2	65	30	15	5	60	
Labium oris	1.0					70	Contact therapy 90 %
Testis	0.3	85	70	25	5	70	

Lit.: 1. EICHHORN, H.J. et al.: Strahlenther. <u>131</u>, 227 (1966)
      2. BARTH, G., BECKER, J.: Klinische Radiologie, Stuttgart,
         New York: Schattauer-Verlag 1968
      3. FLETCHER, G.H.: Textbook of Radiotherapy, Philadelphia:
         Lea and Febiger 1973
      4. OESER, H.: Krebsbekämpfung..., Stuttgart: Thieme 1974

8.9   Typical dose values in biology and medicine
       Typische Dosiswerte in Biologie und Medizin
       Valeurs de dose typiques en biologie et en médecine
       Valores típicos de dosis en biología y medicina

       Average values - Richtwerte - Valeurs moyennes -
       Valores aproximados

1. Smallest dose for which a biologic effect was observed [1]
   Kleinste Dosis, bei der ein biologischer Effekt be-
   obachtet wurde
   Plus petite dose pour laquelle un effet biologique a
   été observé
   Dosis mínima con la que se observa un efecto biológico   5 mrad

2. Dose which kills 1-1/e (= 63 %) of all cells (D_0) [2]
   Dosis, die 1-1/e (= 63 %) aller Zellen abtötet (D_0)
   Dose tuant 1-1/e (= 63 %) de toutes les cellules (D_0)
   Dosis que mata el 1-1/e (= 63 %) de todas las células (D_0)

       Ca cells in vitro - Ca-Zellen in vitro - Cellules
       cancereuses in vitro -Células cancerosas en vitro 100-200   rad

       Cells of root tips in beans - Wurzelspitzen-Zellen
       von Bohnen - Cellules de pointes de racines de fèves
       Células en las puntas de las raices en habas   1000   rad

       Escherichia coli bacteria   10 krad

       Yeast cells (Saccharomyces cerevisiae)   30 krad

       Viruses and bacteriophages   100 krad

3. D_0 for various cells of the living mouse
   D_0 für verschiedene Zellen der lebenden Maus
   D_0 pour différentes cellules de la souris in vivo
   D_0 de varias células de ratones, vivos

       Oocytes   5   rad

       Spermatogonia   180   rad

       Bone marrow stem cells   70   rad

       Intestinal crypt cells   200   rad

4. Suppression of germination in potatoes [3]
   Unterdrückung der Keimfähigkeit von Kartoffeln
   Arrèt de la germination des pommes de terre
   Supresión de la germinación en patatas   8-15 krad

5. Usual sterilising dose for medical products [4]
   Gebräuchliche Sterilisationsdosis für medizinische Erzeugnisse
   Dose stérilisante usuel pour des produits medicaux
   Dosis usual de esterilización, productos medicinales   1-3 Mrad

6. Human skin - Menschliche Haut - Peau humaine -
   Piel humana

       Epilation-transitory   >400   rad

       Epilation-irreversible   >800   rad

       Erythema (see page - siehe Seite - voir page -
       ver página 199)   800   rad

       Radiodermatitis exsudativa   1200   rad

Necrosis	2000	rad
Tolerance dose (field 100 cm^2)	1 x 1700	rad
Idem fractionated: 10 x /14 d =	3700	rad
Idem fractionated: 30 x /42 d =	5500	rad

7. Tolerance doses of different human organs (resulting damage) - Toleranzdosen verschiedener menschlicher Organe und (entstehende Schäden) - Dose de tolerance pour différents organes humains (l'esion résultante) - Dosis de tolerancia para diferentes órganos humanos (resultado del daño) [5]

Fractionated irradiation with 200 rad/d in the organ
Fraktionierte Bestrahlung mit 200 rad/d im Organ
Irradiation fractionnée avec 200 rads/d dans l'organe
Irradiación fraccionada con 200 rad/d en el órgano

Ren (Nephrosklerosis)	2300	rad
Hepar (Budd-Chiari)	3500	rad
Pulmones (Pneumonitis, Fibrosis)	4000	rad
Cerebrum (Necrosis)	5000	rad
Medulla spinalis (Myelitis)	5000	rad
Colon-rectum (Fistula, Stenosis)	5500	rad
Vesica uriniaris (Fistula, Fibrosis)	6000	rad
Os (Necrosis)	6000	rad
Cor (Myocarditis)	4000	rad
Lens (Cataracta)	500	rad
Testis (Azoospermia)	>500	rad
Ovarium (Menolysis)	>200	rad

8. Curative doses frequently used in therapy - in der Therapie zu kurativen Zwecken häufig verabreichte Herddosen Doses curatives fréquemment utilisées en radiothérapie Dosis frecuentemente utilizadas en terapia con fines curativos (Fractionated - Fraktioniert - Fractionnement Fraccionada 200 rad/d)

Seminoma	3000	rad
Lymphogranulomatosis (M. Hodgkin)	4000	rad
Carcinoma laryngis	> 6000	rad
Carcinoma mammae (post operationem)	4000-6000	rad
Osteosarcoma	> 7000	rad
Melanoma (fractionated: 300-1000 rad/d)	< 10-(20)	krad
Arthritis - Arthrosis etc. 5-10·10-20 rad (2/7 d)	50-200	rad

Lit.: 1. FORSSBERG, A.G.: Acta Radiol., Suppl. 49 (1943)
   2. HOFMANN, E.G.: Rö.Prax. 23, 59 (1970)
   3. CHADWICK, K.H.: Proc. IAEA Symp.Dos.Agriculture, Vienna 1973
   4. HUG, O.: Med.Strahlenkunde, Berlin: Springer 1974
   5. RUBIN, P., KELLER, B., QUICK, R. in: The Biological and Clinical Basis of Radiosensitivity, Springfield: Thomas 1974

8.10   Grid or sieve therapy - Gitter- oder Siebbestrahlung - Radiothérapie à travers grilles - Irradiación con rejilla

8.10.1   Explanatory remarks - Erläuterungen - Explications - Explicaciones

The "grid factor" f indicates how the surface dose administered through a grid can be increased compared to that irradiating an open field, while the skin tolerance remains unchanged. The factor increases as the relative aperture Ψ (Ψ = apertures/total field) and the size of the grid holes decrease.

The degree of homogeneity Q is the ratio of the dose under the shielded portions of the field to the dose under the exposed parts of the field. To find the "effectiveness" η of the grid irradiation, i.e., the possible increase in the mean depth dose, one multiplies the grid factor by the relative aperture; i.e.:

$$\eta = f \cdot \Psi.$$

Der "Gitterfaktor" f gibt an, wie die über ein Gitter verabreichte Oberflächendosis gegenüber der auf ein offenes Feld eingestrahlten unter Einhaltung der Hauttoleranz erhöht werden kann. Er wächst mit kleiner werdendem Öffnungsverhältnis Ψ (Ψ = Gitteröffnungen/Gesamtfeld) und mit kleiner werdender Größe der Gitteröffnungen.

Der Homogenitätsgrad Q ist das Verhältnis der Dosis unter den abgedeckten Feldpartien zur Dosis unter den offenen Feldteilen. Der "Wirkungsgrad" η der Gitterbestrahlung, das ist die mögliche Erhöhung der mittleren Tiefendosis, ergibt sich durch Multiplikation des Gitterfaktors mit dem Öffnungsverhältnis, d.h. es ist

$$\eta = f \cdot \Psi.$$

Le "facteur de grille" f représente le facteur par lequel on peutt multiplier la dose à la surface délivrée avec une grille par rapport à celle délivrée par un champ simple sans que la tolérance cutanée soit modifiée. Le facteur augmente lorsque le rapport d'ouverture Ψ (Ψ = surface ouverte de la grille/surface totale du champ) et la taille des trous de la grille diminuent.

Le "coefficient d'homogénéité" Q est le rapport de la dose dans les zônes protegées à la dose dans les zônes irradiées. L'"efficacité" de la grille η, c'est à dire l'accroissement possible de la dose en profondeur s'obtient en multipliant le facteur de grille par le rapport d'ouverture:

$$\eta = f \cdot \Psi.$$

El "factor de rejilla" f indica hasta que punto se puede elevar una dosis superficial suministrada sobre una rejilla, frente a un campo abierto irradiado, manteniendo la tolerancia de piel. El factor aumenta cuando la relación de abertura Ψ (Ψ = aberturas/campo total) y el tamaño de los agujeros de la rejilla disminuye.

El grado de homogeneidad Q es la razón de la dosis bajo la porción blindada del campo a la dosis bajo las partes expuestas del campo. Para encontrar la "efectividad" η de la irradiación con rejilla, esto es el aumento posible en la dosis de profundidad media, se multiplica el factor de rejilla por la abertura relativa; esto es:

$$\eta = f \cdot \Psi.$$

Lit.: 1. LOEVINGER, R., WOLF, B.S., MINOWITZ, W.: Am.J.Roentgenol. 64, 999 (1950)
    2. COHEN, O.A., PALAZZO, W.L.: Am.J.Roentgenol. 67, 470 (1952)
    3. LOEVINGER, R.: Radiology 58, 351 (1952)
    4. JOLLES, B., MITCHELL, R.G.: Brit.J.Radiol. 27, 407 (1954)

8.10.2   <u>Practical values for f, η, and Q</u>
          <u>Praktische Werte für f, η und Q</u>
          <u>Valeurs pratiques pour f, η et Q</u>
          <u>Valores prácticos para f, η, y Q</u>

8.10.2.1 <u>Grid factors - Gitterfaktoren - Facteurs de grille -</u>
          <u>Factores de rejilla (f)</u>

Valid for 200 kV= (≈ 1.7 mm Cu HVL); field size ∿100 cm^2
and grid holes of about 10 mm diameter - Gültig für
200 kV= (≈ 1,7 mm Cu HWSD), Feldgrößen von ∿100 cm^2 und
Gitteröffnungen von 10 mm Durchmesser - Valable pour:
200 kV= (≈ 1,7 mm Cu CHA); champs de 100 cm^2 et diametres
des ouvertures de la grille 10 mm - Válido para: 200 kV=
(≈ 1,7 mm Cu CHR); campos de 100 cm^2 y aberturas de la
rejilla de 10 mm diámetro

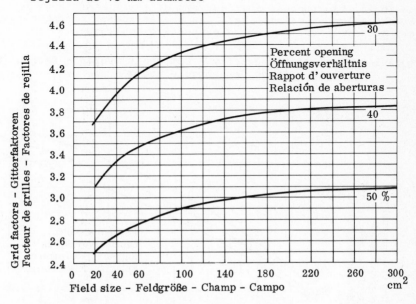

Field	Grid factors - Gitterfaktoren - Facteurs de grille - Factores de rejilla and - und - et - y					f
Feld	Effectivness - Wirkungsgrad - Efficacité - Efectividad					η
Champ	Percent opening - Öffnungsverhältnis - Rapport d'ouverture - Relación de aberturas					%
Campo	30		40		50	
cm^2	f	η	f	η	f	η
20	3.70	1.10	3.10	1.24	2.50	1.25
40	3.95	1.18	3.35	1.34	2.65	1.33
60	4.15	1.24	3.45	1.38	2.75	1.37
80	4.25	1.27	3.55	1.42	3.25	1.43
100	4.35	1.30	3.60	1.44	2.90	1.45
150	4.45	1.34	3.75	1.49	3.00	1.50
200	4.55	1.36	3.80	1.51	3.05	1.53
250	4.60	1.38	3.80	1.53	3.05	1.54
300	4.60	1.39	3.85	1.54	3.10	1.55

Note - Bemerkung - Remarque - Nota:

For fractionated doses the grid factors (f) are optimal (= maximal)
only if the grids are applied in such a way that the same skin areas
are always exposed or protected respectively.

Die Gitterfaktoren (f) sind bei fraktionierter Dosisverabreichung nur
dann optimal (= maximal), wenn die Gitter immer so aufgelegt werden,
daß jedesmal die gleichen Hautstellen offen bzw. abgedeckt sind.

Pour les irradiations fractionnées les facteurs de grille (f) sont
maxima seulement si la grille est mise en place de telle façon que
ce soient les mêmes surfaces de peau qui soient toujours irradiées
ou protegées.

Para dosis fraccionadas los factores de rejilla (f) son optimos (=
maximal) solamente si las rejillas son aplicadas en forma tal, que la
misma área de piel es siempre expuesta o desligada.

8.10.2.2 Degree of homogeneity - Homogenitätsgrad - Degré d'homo-généité - Grado de homogeneidad *)

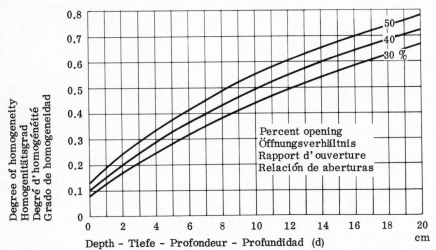

Depth - Tiefe - Profondeur - Profundidad (d)

*) Definition homogeneity see page - Begriff Homogenität siehe
Seite - Définition d'homogénéité voir page - Definición homogeneidad ver página 208

d cm	Degree of homogeneity - Homogenitätsgrad - Degré d'homo-généité - Grado de homogeneidad Ω			d cm			%
	ψ				ψ		
	30	40	50		30	40	50
0	0.08	0.10	0.13	8	0.38	0.43	0.48
1	0.13	0.15	0.18	10	0.44	0.48	0.55
2	0.17	0.20	0.24	12	0.50	0.55	0.60
3	0.21	0.24	0.28	14	0.55	0.60	0.65
4	0.24	0.28	0.33	16	0.60	0.65	0.70
5	0.27	0.33	0.37	18	0.65	0.70	0.75
6	0.32	0.37	0.42	20	0.70	0.75	0.80

Table of contents - Inhaltsverzeichnis
Table des matières - Tabla de materias

9.1 Dose limits for man – Dosisgrenzwerte für Personen
Limites de dose pour les individus – Dosis limites para individuos

Organ / Organ / Organe / Organo	Occupationally exposed persons / Beruflich Strahlenexponierte / Travailleurs professionnellement exposés / Ocupacionalmente expuesto		Individual member of the public / Einzelpersonen der Bevölkerung / Individu donné de la population / Individuos de la población en general	General population / Gesamtbevölkerung / Population / Población
	rem/a	rem/1/4 a	rem/a	rem/30 a
Gonads, red bone marrow, whole body / Gonaden, rotes Knochenmark, Ganzkörper / Gonades, moelle rouge, corps entier / Ganados, médula roja, cuerpo total	5	3	0.5	5
Skin, thyroid gland, bone / Haut, Schilddrüse, Knochen / Peau, thyroïde, os / Piel, glándula tiroidea, hueso	30	15	3(1.5)	
Hands, forearms, feet, ankles / Hände, Unterarme, Füße, Knöchel / Mains, avant-bras, pieds, chevilles / Manos, antebrazos, pies, tobillos	75	40	7.5	
All other organs individually / Alle anderen Organe einzeln / Tout les autres organes individuellement / Todos los demás órganos	15	8	1.5	

For a full discussion of dose limits the reader is referred to:
Einzelheiten sind aus folgenden Publikationen zu entnehmen:
Pour une discussion complète sur les limites de dose, le
lecteur est renvoyé à:
Para mayores detalles remitimos al lector a las publicaciones:

ICRP Publ. 9(1966), 2(1967), 10(1968)
22(1973). Oxford: Pergamon Press
IAEA Safety Series No. 9 (1967)
ENEA Radiation Protection Norms 1968
NCRP Report 39, Washington 1971

9.2 Important activities and concentrations (soluble substances)
Wichtige Aktivitäten und Konzentrationen (lösliche Stoffe)
Activités et concentrations notables (matériaux solubles)
Actividades y concentraciones importantes (material solubles)

Nuclide Nuklid Nucléide Nuclido	1 μCi	2 *) μCi	3 *) μCi	4 *) μCi/cm³	5 **) a μCi	5 **) b μCi	6 a rem/μCi	6 b rem/μCi
^{51}Cr	100	800	$2.7 \cdot 10^4$	$4 \cdot 10^{-6}$	$1.3 \cdot 10^3$	$2.7 \cdot 10^3$	$1.2 \cdot 10^{-3}$	$3.3 \cdot 10^{-4}$
^{57}Co	10	200	$8.7 \cdot 10^3$	$5 \cdot 10^{-3}$	$4.3 \cdot 10^2$	$8.7 \cdot 10^2$	$3.6 \cdot 10^{-3}$	$5.5 \cdot 10^{-4}$
^{58}Co	10	30	$2.4 \cdot 10^3$	$3 \cdot 10^{-7}$	$1.0 \cdot 10^2$	$2.4 \cdot 10^2$	$1.5 \cdot 10^{-2}$	$2.4 \cdot 10^{-3}$
^{59}Fe	10	20	$3.7 \cdot 10^2$	$5 \cdot 10^{-8}$	$4.7 \cdot 10^2$	$3.7 \cdot 10$	$3.3 \cdot 10^{-2}$	$4.0 \cdot 10^{-2}$
^{75}Se	10	90	$3.1 \cdot 10^3$	$4 \cdot 10^{-7}$	$2.4 \cdot 10^2$	$3.1 \cdot 10^2$	$6.3 \cdot 10^{-3}$	$5.0 \cdot 10^{-3}$
^{85}Sr	10	60	$5.8 \cdot 10^2$	$8 \cdot 10^{-8}$	$7.6 \cdot 10$	$5.8 \cdot 10$	$1.3 \cdot 10^{-2}$	$3.0 \cdot 10^{-2}$
^{99m}Tc	100	200	$9.5 \cdot 10^4$	10^{-5}	$4.6 \cdot 10^3$	$9.5 \cdot 10^3$	$(3 \cdot 10^{-4})$	$(1.5 \cdot 10^{-4})$
^{113m}In	100	30	$2.1 \cdot 10^4$	$3 \cdot 10^{-6}$	$1.0 \cdot 10^3$	$2.1 \cdot 10^3$	$(5 \cdot 10^{-4})$	$(2.0 \cdot 10^{-4})$
^{125}I	(1)	(1)	$(4 \cdot 10)$	$(5 \cdot 10^{-9})$	(2.4)	(4.0)	(1.2)	(0.75)
^{131}I	1	0.7	$2.1 \cdot 10$	$(3 \cdot 10^{-9})$	1.6	2.1	2.0	1.6
^{132}I	10	0.3	$5.9 \cdot 10^2$	$(8 \cdot 10^{-8})$	4.5	$5.9 \cdot 10$	$6 \cdot 10^{-2}$	$4.5 \cdot 10^{-2}$
^{137}Cs	10	30	$1.6 \cdot 10^2$	$2 \cdot 10^{-8}$	$1.2 \cdot 10$	$1.6 \cdot 10$	$1.1 \cdot 10^{-1}$	$8 \cdot 10^{-2}$
^{197}Hg	100	20	$2.9 \cdot 10^3$	$4 \cdot 10^{-7}$	$2.4 \cdot 10^2$	$2.9 \cdot 10^2$	$5.2 \cdot 10^{-3}$	$4.5 \cdot 10^{-3}$
^{198}Au	10	20	$8 \cdot 10^2$	10^{-7}	$4.1 \cdot 10$	$8 \cdot 10$	$3.4 \cdot 10^{-2}$	$2.6 \cdot 10^{-4}$
^{203}Hg	10	4	$1.8 \cdot 10^2$	$2 \cdot 10^{-8}$	$1.4 \cdot 10$	$1.8 \cdot 10$	$1.0 \cdot 10^{-1}$	$8 \cdot 10^{-2}$

1. Maximum permissible activity for exemption from notification, registration or licensing - Freigrenze - Activité maximale permettant l'exemption de la déclaration où de la demande d'agréement - Limite de libertad

2. Maximum permissible total body burden - Höchstzugelassene Körperaktivität - Activité corporelle maximale permissible - Carga corporal máxima permisible

3. Maximum permissible annual intake by inhalation during working hours - Maximal zulässige Jahresaktivitätszufuhr über die Luft während der Arbeitszeit - Quantité inhalée maximale permissible durant des heures de travail - Aporte de carga anual máximo permisible por inhalación durante las horas de trabajo

4. Maximum permissible concentration in inhaled air; exposure time 168 h/week - Maximal zulässige Konzentration in der Atemluft, Einwirkungsdauer 168 h/Woche - Concentration maximale permissible pour l'air inhalé; temps de référence: 168 h/semaine - Concentración máxima permisible en el aire inhalado, tiempo de influencia 168 h/semana

5. Limiting value for annual intake by (a) ingestion and (b) inhalation - Grenzwert der Jahresaktivitäszufuhr durch (a) Ingestion und (b) Inhalation - Valeurs limites des quantités annuelles a) ingérée et b) inhalée - Valores límites del aporte de carga anual por a) ingestión b) inhalación

6. Dose commitment (50 a), single intake - Folge-Äquivalentdosis (50 a), einmalige Aufnahme - Dose engagée (50 a), incorporation unique - Dosis sucesiva, equivalente (50 a), toma unica

*) Workers - Arbeiter - Travailleurs - Trabajadores
**) Member of the public - Einzelperson der Bevölkerung - Individu de la population Individuo de la población

Lit.: See page - Siehe Seite - Voir page - Ver página 212

9.3 Mean doses to the whole body, gonads or organs
Mittlere Ganzkörper-, Gonaden- oder Organdosen
Doses moyennes délivrées à l'ensemble de l'organisme, aux
gonades ou aux différents organes
Doses medianos a cuerpo entero, gónados or órganos

(Maximal values neglected - Höchstwerte vernachlässigt - Les valeurs
extrêmes n'ont pas été retenues - Valores maximales desuidos)

		min.	mrad/a mean	max.
1. Natural sources - Natürliche Strahlenquellen - Sources naturelles - Fuentes naturales				
1.1 Cosmic radiation - Kosmische Strahlung - 0 m		20	30	40
Rayonnement cosmique - Rayos cósmicos 1000 m		30	40	50
1.2 Terestrial radiation - Umgebungsstrahlung Rayonnement terrestre - Radiación terrestral		20	45	150
(Maximum values - Höchstwerte - Valeurs maximales - Valores máximos Kerala/India, Guarapari/Brazil		-	∿1000	>3000)
1.3 Incorporated radionuclides - Inkorporierte Radionuklide - Radionucléides dans le corps humain - Radionúclidos incorporados)		10	20	40
1.4 Additional radiation in houses - Zusätzliche Strahlung in Gebäuden - Irradiations additionelles dues aux bâtiments - Radiación adicional en las casas		<0	15	30
Total - Zusammen - Total - Total		∿60	∿110	∿270

2. Artificial sources - Künstliche Strahlenquellen
Sources d'origine humaine - Fuentes artificiales

	min.	mean	max.
2.1 Medicine - Medizin - Médecine - Medicina Total:	20	50	80
2.1.1 Diagnosis - Diagnostik - Diagnóstic - Diagnóstico	16	48	76
2.1.2 Therapy - Therapie - Thérapie - Terapía	0.5	1	2
2.1.3 Nuclear medicine - Nuklearmedizin - Médecine nucléaire - Medicina nuclear	0.5	1	2
2.2 Occupational exposure - Berufliche Strahlenbelastung - Exposition professionnelle - Exposición ocupacional		<1	
2.3 Radioactivity in consumer goods - Radioaktivität in Verbrauchsgütern - Radioactivité des biens de consommation - Radiactividad en los productos del consumidor	1	2	4
2.4 Fall·out - Fall out - Retombées - Lluvia radiactiva	3	4	10
2.5 Nuclear power plants - Kernkraftwerke - Centrales nucléaires - Plantas nucleares		< 1	
Total - Zusammen - Total - Total	∿25	∿60	∿100

9.4 Components of cosmic radiation at various altitudes
Komponenten der kosmischen Strahlung in verschiedenen Höhen
Composants du rayonnement cosmique à diverses altitudes
Componentes de radiación cósmica a diferentes altitudes

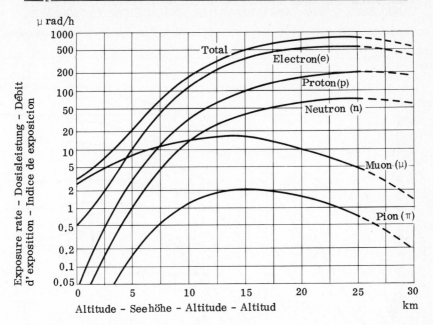

Altitude Seehöhe Altitude Altitud	Exposure rate - Dosisleistung - Débit d'exposition - Indice de exposición µrad/h					
	Particle - Teilchen - Particules - Partículas					
km	π	µ	n	p	e⁻	total
0	(<0.01)	2.7	(0.015)	0.04	0.5	3.2
1	(<0.01)	3.4	0.04	0.12	0.8	4.3
2	(<0.01)	4.2	0.1	0.3	1.4	6.0
3	0.04	5.2	0.25	0.7	2.8	9.0
4	0.08	6.5	0.5	1.5	5.4	14
5	0.15	8.0	1.0	3.0	10	22
7.5	0.35	12	4.4	12	40	69
10	1.2	14	14	34	110	173
12.5	1.8	16	26	60	220	324
15	2.0	15	35	100	360	512
17.5	1.9	13	50	135	450	650
20	1.6	10	62	165	500	740
22.5	1.1	7.0	68	190	550	820
25	0.7	4.5	73	200	550	830
27.5	(0.4)	(2.7)	(65)	(195)	(480)	(750)
30	(0.2)	(1.3)	(58)	(170)	(370)	(600)

Lit.: 1. ICRP Publ. 18, Oxford: Pergamon Press 1972

215

Average half- and tenth-value layers of shielding materials
Mittlere Halb- und Zehntelwertschichten von Abschirmstoffen
Couches moyennes de demi atténuation et d'atténuation 1/10
pour les matériaux utilisés en radioprotection
Capas hemi y deci reductoras para materiales de blindaje

Broad beams - Breite Felder - Champs larges - Campos anchos

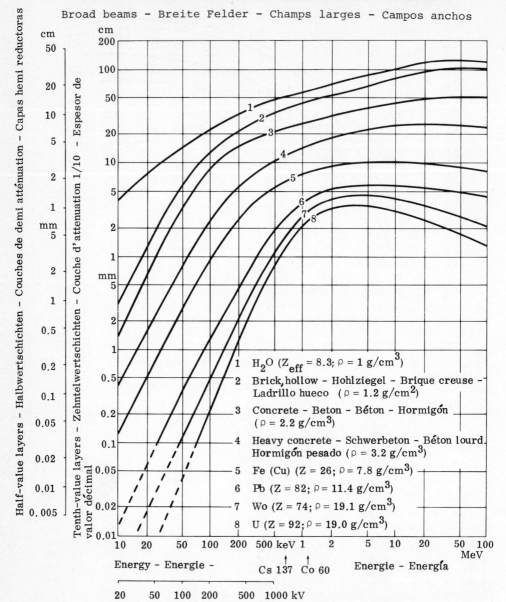

Left axis labels:
Half-value layers – Halbwertschichten – Couches de demi atténuation – Capas hemi reductoras
Tenth-value layers – Zehntelwertschichten – Couche d'attenuation 1/10 – Espesor de valor decimal

Legend:

1 H_2O (Z_{eff} = 8.3; ρ = 1 g/cm^3)

2 Brick, hollow - Hohlziegel - Brique creuse - Ladrillo hueco (ρ = 1.2 g/cm^2)

3 Concrete - Beton - Béton - Hormigón (ρ = 2.2 g/cm^3)

4 Heavy concrete - Schwerbeton - Béton lourd. Hormigón pesado (ρ = 3.2 g/cm^3)

5 Fe (Cu) (Z = 26; ρ = 7.8 g/cm^3)

6 Pb (Z = 82; ρ = 11.4 g/cm^3)

7 Wo (Z = 74; ρ = 19.1 g/cm^3)

8 U (Z = 92; ρ = 19.0 g/cm^3)

Energy - Energie -   Cs 137   Co 60   Energie - Energía

Tube voltage - Röhrenspannung - Tension d'alimentation - Voltaje del tubo

Energy Energie Energie Energía	HVL - HWSD - CDA - CHR (Rounded values - Abgerundete Zahlenwerte - Valeurs arrondies - Valores redondeados)								
E	Material - Stoff - Matériau - Material								
	1 (H_2O)	2	3	4	5 (Fe)	6 (Pb)	7 (W)	8 *) (U)	
10 keV	1.2	0.9	0.4	0.12	0.04	(0.004)	–	–	mm
20	2.3	3.9	1.4	0.5	0.16	(0.009)	(0.006)	–	
50	4.2	1.7	1.0	2.3	0.8	0.11	0.035	(0.012)	
100	6.8	3.8	2.5	7.0	2.7	0.38	0.14	0.065	
200	10	6.5	4.4	1.7	7.3	1.35	0.65	0.38	
500	14	10	6.4	3.1	1.6	5.6	3.2	2.3	
Cs 137	15	11	6.8	3.5	1.8	7.0	4.5	3.4	
1 MeV	16	12	7.5	4.2	2.2	1.1	7.8	6.1	cm
Co 60	17	14	8.0	4.5	2.4	1.2	9.0	7.2	
2	20	15	9.2	5.4	2.7	1.6	1.2	1.0	
5	23	19	11	6.7	3.0	1.7	1.3	1.0	
10	28	22	13	7.2	3.0	1.7	1.2	0.9	
20	35	28	14	7.6	3.0	1.6	1.0	0.7	
50	38	31	15	7.3	2.6	1.4	0.8	0.5	
100	35	30	15	7.0	2.4	1.3	0.63	0.38	
E	1/10 VL - 1/10 WSD - CA 1/10 - C 1/10 R								
10 keV	3.8	3.2	1.4	0.4	0.13	(0.013)	–	–	mm
20	7.6	1.3	6.5	1.7	0.55	(0.06)	(0.018)	–	
50	15	6.0	3.5	8.0	2.7	0.38	0.11	0.04	
100	23	13	9.0	2.4	9.0	1.3	0.45	0.22	
200	34	22	15	5.7	2.6	4.7	2.2	1.3	
500	48	35	22	11	5.5	2.0	1.1	8	
Cs 137	52	39	24	12	6.4	2.8	1.8	1.3	
1 MeV	58	50	26	15	7.6	3.8	2.8	2.2	cm
Co 60	60	51	28	16	7.9	4.0	3.1	2.4	
2	70	54	33	18	9.4	5.5	4.2	3.3	
5	87	66	38	23	10	5.8	4.6	3.5	
10	100	78	44	25	11	5.8	4.2	3.0	
20	120	96	48	26	10	5.5	3.5	2.4	
50	122	104	50	25	8.6	4.9	2.7	1.8	
100	120	103	50	23	8.0	4.4	2.1	1.3	

*) Numbers 1 - 8 see page 216
Zahlen 1 - 8 vergl. Kurven auf Seite 216
Pour les numeros 1 - 8 voir page 216
Cifras 1 - 8 ver página 216

Lit.: 1. GLADYS, WHITE, R.: NBS-Report No. 1003 (1952)
2. LORENTZON, L.: Acta Radiol. 41, 201 (1954)
3. NCRP Report No. 33 (1968)
4. ICRP Report No. 21 (1971)
5. MARUYAMA, R. et al.: Hlth. Phys. 20, 277 (1971)
6. JAEGER, R., HÜBNER, W.: Dosimetrie und Strahlenschutz, Stuttgart: Thieme 1974
7. TROUT, D.E. et al.: Hlth. Phys. 29, 163 (1975)

9.6   Transmission of rays through shielding walls
        Durchlässigkeit von Abschirmwänden für Strahlungen
        Transmission des rayonnements à travers des écrans protecteurs
        Permeabilidad de las radiaciones a través de blindaje

9.6.1   50 - 300 kV X-rays - Röntgenstrahlen - Rayons X - Rayos X

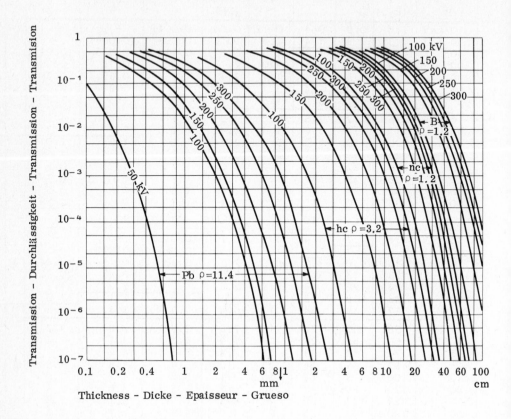

Thickness - Dicke - Epaisseur - Grueso

Pb (ρ = 11.35) = Lead - Blei - Plomb - Plomo

hc (ρ = 3.2) = Heavy concrete - Schwerbeton - Béton lourd - Hormigón
                pesado

nc (ρ = 2.2) = Normal concrete - Normalbeton - Béton normal -
                Hormigón normal

B (ρ = 1.2) = Brick - Ziegel - Brique - Ladrillo

kV = Normal radiation - Normalstrahlung - Rayonnement normal -
    Radiación normal

Lit.: 1. ICRP, Suppl. 15, Oxford (1970)
     2. KELLEY, J.P., TROUT, E.D.: Radiology 104, 171 (1972)
     3. DIN 6812, Berlin: Beuth-Verlag, Februar 1974
     4. Authors' measurements - Eigene Messungen - Mesures perso-
       nelles - Medidas propias

Required thickness - Erforderliche Abschirmung - Epaisseur nécessaire - Espesor requerido   mm, cm

With tube voltages - Bei Röhrenspannungen - Tension du tube - Con tensión del tubo   kV

Transmission Durchlässigkeit Transmission Transmisión	Lead - Blei Plomb - Plomo (mm)						Heavy concrete - Barytbeton Béton baryté-Hormigón pesado (cm)					
	kV 50	100	150	200	250	300	kV 50	100	150	200	250	300
10^{-1}	0.10	0.45	0.62	1.0	1.4	2.0	(0.09)	0.35	0.90	1.8	2.9	3.4
$5 \cdot 10^{-2}$	0.12	0.65	0.86	1.3	2.0	3.0	(0.13)	0.5	1.3	2.4	3.5	4.6
10^{-2}	0.17	1.1	1.5	2.2	3.5	5.0	(0.26)	1.0	2.4	4.1	6.1	7.8
$5 \cdot 10^{-3}$	0.20	1.4	1.8	2.7	4.2	6.3	(0.31)	1.2	3.0	5.0	7.2	9.0
10^{-3}	0.27	2.0	2.5	3.6	6.0	9.0	(0.44)	1.7	4.0	6.7	9.8	12
$5 \cdot 10^{-4}$	0.30	2.3	2.8	4.2	6.7	10	(0.49)	1.9	4.6	7.7	11	14
10^{-4}	0.36	3.1	3.5	5.6	8.7	14	(0.65)	2.5	6.0	9.5	14	17
$5 \cdot 10^{-5}$	0.40	3.3	4.0	6.1	9.8	15	(0.70)	2.7	6.4	11	15	18
10^{-5}	0.45	4.3	5.0	7.8	12	17	(0.80)	3.1	7.9	13	18	22
$5 \cdot 10^{-6}$	0.48	4.7	5.4	8.3	13	19	(0.85)	3.3	8.5	14	23	23
10^{-6}	0.54	5.5	6.2	9.9	15	22	(0.98)	3.8	10	16	22	27
$5 \cdot 10^{-7}$	0.57	5.7	6.7	10.5	16	24	(1.04)	4.0	10.5	17	23	28
10^{-7}	0.62	6.0	7.3	12	18	28	(1.14)	4.4	11.5	19	26	31

	Concrete - Beton Béton - Hormigón (cm)						Brick - Ziegel Brique - Ladrillo (cm)					
	kV 50	100	150	200	250	300	kV 50	100	150	200	250	300
10^{-1}	1.3	4.3	7.3	9.2	10.5	13	3.5	13	18	21	23	25
$5 \cdot 10^{-2}$	1.7	5.6	9.4	12	14	15	4.3	16	22	25	27	30
10^{-2}	2.7	9.0	15	18	20	21	6.2	23	30	35	39	43
$5 \cdot 10^{-3}$	3.2	10.5	17	20	22	22	6.7	25	34	38	44	48
10^{-3}	4.5	15	21	26	29	27	8.5	32	43	49	54	60
$5 \cdot 10^{-4}$	5.1	17	23	29	31	31	9.0	34	46	53	60	64
10^{-4}	6.0	20	28	34	36	36	11	42	53	64	69	75
$5 \cdot 10^{-5}$	6.6	22	30	36	40	37	12	43	56	67	74	(80)
10^{-5}	7.8	26	34	41	46	43	14	50	66	80	-	-
$5 \cdot 10^{-6}$	8.4	28	36	43	50	46	15	54	69	(85)	-	-
10^{-6}	9.3	31	42	50	47	51	17	61	80	-	-	-
$5 \cdot 10^{-7}$	9.5	32	44	52	60	54	17	63	(85)	-	-	-
10^{-7}	10.0	34	48	59	66	60	19	70	-	-	-	-

<u>I 131, Cs 137, Co 60, 5 - 100 MV</u>

<u>X- and gamma rays - Röntgen- und Gammastrahlen - Rayons X et</u>
<u>rayons gamma - Rayos X y gamma</u>

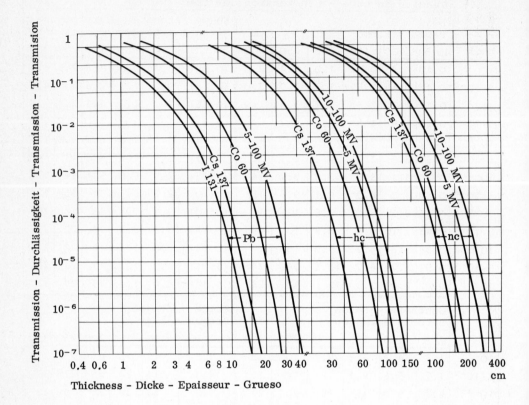

Thickness - Dicke - Epaisseur - Grueso

Pb (ρ = 11.35) = Lead - Blei - Plomb - Plomo

hc (ρ = 3.2) = Heavy concrete - Schwerbeton - Béton lourd - Hormigón
pesado

nc (ρ = 2.2) = Normal concrete - Normalbeton - Béton normal -
Hormigón normal

I 131 = γ-radiation of ^{131}I (E = 640 keV) - γ-Strahlung von ^{131}J

(E = 640 keV) - Radiation γ de ^{131}I (E = 640 keV) - Radiación

γ de ^{131}I (E = 640 keV)

Lit.: 1. MARUYAMA, T. et al.: Health Phys. <u>20</u>, 277 (1971)
2. SAUERMANN, D.F., FRIEDRICH, W., MITLACHER, H.: Tagungsbe-
richte, Fachverband für Strahlenschutz, 241 (1973)

Transmission / Durchlässigkeit / Transmission / Transmisión	Required thickness - Erforderliche Abschirmung - Epaisseur nécessaire - Espesor requerido mm, cm											
	With γ-radiation of - Bei γ-Strahlungen von - Avec rayonnement γ de - Con radiación γ de kV											
	Lead - Blei / Plomb - Plomo mm				Heavy concrete / Barytbeton / Béton baryte / Hormigón pesado cm				Concrete / Beton / Béton / Hormigón cm			
	^{131}I	Cs	Co	5-100 MV	Cs	Co	5 MV	10-100 MV	Cs	Co	5 MV	10-100 MV
$5 \cdot 10^{-1}$	0.46	0.67	1.3	1.9	2.7	4.3	6.6	7.5	7.0	8.5	13	16
$2 \cdot 10^{-1}$	1.0	1.4	2.8	4.5	5.3	8.8	12	14	15	18	26	34
10^{-1}	1.7	2.1	4.2	6.6	7.6	12	17	19	22	26	37	48
$5 \cdot 10^{-2}$	2.1	2.8	5.2	8.0	9.8	17	21	25	28	34	49	63
$2 \cdot 10^{-2}$	3.0	3.9	6.9	11	13	22	28	32	37	46	63	82
10^{-2}	3.7	4.8	8.1	13	15	25	33	39	42	52	74	96
$5 \cdot 10^{-3}$	4.4	5.7	9.4	15	18	28	38	47	50	60	85	110
$2 \cdot 10^{-3}$	5.3	6.8	11	17	21	33	45	52	58	70	104	130
10^{-3}	6.0	7.5	13	19	22	37	50	60	65	80	114	145
$5 \cdot 10^{-4}$	6.7	8.3	14	21	25	41	54	64	71	85	125	160
$2 \cdot 10^{-4}$	7.6	9.4	15	23	28	46	62	72	80	98	140	180
10^{-4}	8.1	10	17	25	30	50	67	80	88	105	150	190
$5 \cdot 10^{-5}$	8.8	11	18	27	32	53	71	85	95	114	160	205
$2 \cdot 10^{-5}$	9.7	12	19	29	36	59	78	94	105	125	180	230
10^{-5}	10.3	12	20	30	38	63	83	103	110	135	190	245
$5 \cdot 10^{-6}$	11	13	22	32	41	67	89	110	115	140	200	260
$2 \cdot 10^{-6}$	12	14	23	34	43	71	96	117	128	155	220	280
10^{-6}	13	15	24	36	46	75	102	123	135	165	240	300
$5 \cdot 10^{-7}$	13	16	25	38	49	79	108	130	140	175	250	315
$2 \cdot 10^{-7}$	14	17	27	40	53	85	112	138	155	180	270	335
10^{-7}	15	18	28	42	55	89	120	145	160	190	275	350

9.7   <u>Quantity and quality of back-scattered X-radiation</u>
      <u>Quantität und Qualität rückgestreuter Röntgenstrahlung</u>
      <u>Quantité et qualité des rayonnements X rétrodiffusés</u>
      <u>Cantidad y calidad de la radiación dispersa de los rayos X</u>

Conditions of measurement - Meßbedingungen - Conditions de mesure -
Condiciones de medida

20 x 20 cm^2 Field area - Feldgröße - Champ - Campo

50 cm Distance source/scatterer/radiation detector; thick scattering
medium (d > 3 HVL) - Abstand Strahlenquelle/Streukörper/Strahlendetek-
tor; Dicke Streukörper (d > 3 HWSD) - Distance source/milieu diffu-
sant/détecteur; épaisseur de milieu diffusant (d > 3 CDA) - Distancia
fuente/cuerpo disperson/detector; espesor del cuerpo dispersor
(d > 3 CHR)

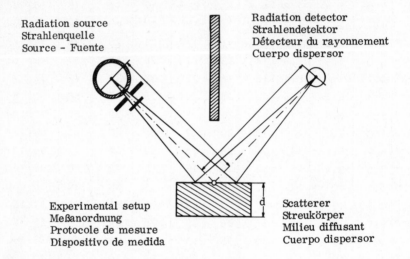

Radiation source   Radiation detector
Strahlenquelle   Strahlendetektor
Source - Fuente   Détecteur du rayonnement
                          Cuerpo dispersor

Experimental setup   Scatterer
Meßanordnung   Streukörper
Protocole de mesure   Milieu diffusant
Dispositivo de medida   Cuerpo dispersor

The data given in the graphs must be regarded as relative only since
they are strongly dependent on the distances and angles between radiation source, scatterer, and detector. Therefore the results are
presented only in graphic form.

Die aus den Kurven ablesbaren Daten müssen relativ betrachtet werden,
da sie stark von den Abständen und Winkeln Strahlenquelle/Streukör-
per/Detektor abhängen. Aus diesem Grunde sind die Ergebnisse nur in
Kurvenform dargestellt.

Les valeurs figurant sur les courbes sont des données approchées,
car elles dépendent beaucoup des distances et des angles entre la
source, le diffuseur et le détecteur. C'est pourquoi les résultats
sont présentés seulement sous une forme graphique.

Los valores mostrados deben considerarse como relativos ya que - los
valores absolutos dependen en gran parte de la distancia y los ángulos
de la fuente/cuerpo dispersor/detector y tamaño del campo irradiado.

Lit.: 1. WACHSMANN, F.: Fortschr.Röntgenstr. <u>101</u>, 308 (1964)
      2. WACHSMANN, F.: Radiologia diagnostica <u>6</u>, 369 (1965)
      3. ICRP <u>21</u>, (1971)

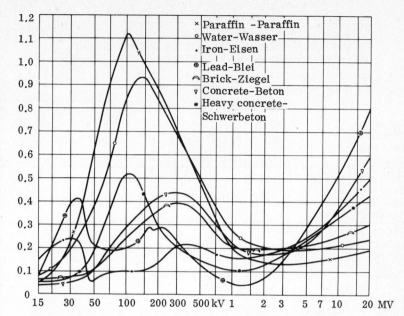

Quantity of scattered radiation/primary radiation
Quantität der gestreuten Strahlung/Primärstrahlung
Quantité de rayonnement rétrodiffusé/primaire
Cantidad de la radiación dispersa/primaria

Legend:
× Paraffin - Paraffin
○ Water-Wasser
. Iron-Eisen
⊕ Lead-Blei
⌒ Brick-Ziegel
▽ Concrete-Beton
✳ Heavy concrete-Schwerbeton

Normal radiation - Normalstrahlung - Rayonnement normal
Radiación normal

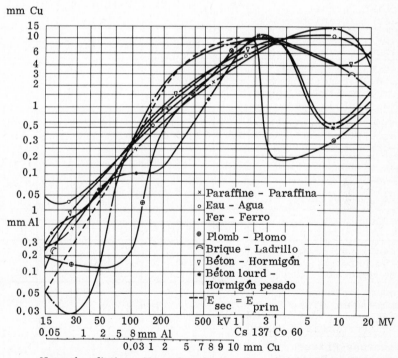

HVL of the scattered radiation - HWSD der gestreuten Strahlung
CDA du rayonnement rétrodiffusé - CHR de la radiación retrodispersa

mm Cu

mm Al

Legend:
× Paraffine - Paraffina
○ Eau - Agua
. Fer - Ferro
⊕ Plomb - Plomo
⌒ Brique - Ladrillo
▽ Béton - Hormigón
✳ Béton lourd - Hormigón pesado
--- $E_{sec} = E_{prim}$

0.05   1   2   5   8 mm Al

Cs 137 Co 60

0.03 1 2   5 7 8 9 10 mm Cu

Normal radiation - Normalstrahlung - Rayonnement normal
Radiación normal

9.8 Radioactivity in building materials
Radioaktivität in Baustoffen
Radioactivité des matériaux de construction
Radioactividad en materiales de construcción

Average values - Richtwerte
Valeurs moyennes - Valores orientativos

Material Material Matériaux Material	Activity - Aktivität - Activité - Actividad nCi/kg								
	^{40}K			^{226}Ra			^{232}Th		
	min.	med.	max.	min.	med.	max.	min.	med.	max.
Sand and gravel Sand und Kies Sable et gravier Arena y grava	0.2	7	18	0.1	<0.4	0.8	0.1	<0.4	1
Other natural stone Andere Natursteine Autres pierres natur. Otras piedras naturales	1	<13	25	0.5	0.7	1.2	0.5	<0.8	1.4
Lava, basalt Tuffstein, Basalt Lave, basalte Toba, basalto	11	38	55	0.4	1.1	2.3	0.2	<0.5	1.4
Slate, granite Schiefer, Granit Ardoise, granit Pizarra, granito	24	40	96	0.8	1.5	3.6	1.1	2.2	5.2
Brick - Ziegel Brique - Ladrillo	4	17	69	0.6	2.2	6.7	0.5	2.6	10
" with 30 % red mud " mit 30 % Rotschlamm " avec 30 % boue rouge " con 30 % de barro rojo		13			5			5	
Pumice - Bimsstein Pierre ponce Piedra pomez	13	24	30	0.7	2.2	3.6	1.1	2.3	4.6
Slag-stone Schlackensteine Scories Piedra de escorias	3	9	16	1.2	2.2	3.2	0.6	2.8	5.6
Cement - Zement Ciment - Cemento	0.5	<4	7	0.3	<1.4	5.3	0.3	<1.4	5.2
Gypsum, nat.-Naturgips Gypse naturel Yeso natural	0.7	2.4	5		<0.7			<0.5	
Gypsum, techn. Technischer Gips Gypse techn. Yeso artificial técnico	0.8	<2	6	7	14	28		<0.5	
Flagstone-Fliesen Carrelage - Baldosas	5	13	31	0.6	1.7	2.7	0.7	1.9	4.9

Lit.: 1. Schmier, H.: Jahresbericht Bundesgesundheitsamt, Berlin
Bundesministerium des Innern 1973

9.9   Typical dose values in radiation protection
        Typische Dosiswerte im Strahlenschutz
        Valeurs des doses typiques en radioprotection
        Valores típicos de dosis en protección

1. Dose limits for the total population and for professionally exposed persons, in whole-body and partial irradiation - Dosisgrenz-
   werte für die Gesamtbevölkerung und die beruflich Strahlenexpo-
   nierten bei Ganz- und Teilkörperbestrahlungen - Limites de dose
   pour l'ensemble de la population et pour les travailleurs profes-
   sionnellement exposés lors d'irradiations totales ou partielles -
   Dosis límites para la población total y para personas afectadas
   de exposición por razones profesionales, radiación corporal total
   y parcial

        See page - Siehe Seite - Voir page - Ver página 212

2. Symptoms following a single total-body exposure
   Symptome bei einmaliger Ganzkörperbestrahlung
   Symptômes suivant une irradiation totale unique
   Síntomas a consecuencia de una exposición unica
   del cuerpo total

        Initial symptoms - Erste Symptome - Symptômes
        initiaux - Primeros síntomas   >50 rad

        Life-threatening radiation sickness - Lebensbedrohliche
        Strahlenkrankheit - Maladie des irradiations menaçant
        la vie - Enfermedad radioactiva con peligro mortal   >200 rad

        50 % lethal dose for man - 50 % Letaldosis/Mensch
        Dose létale 50 % chez l'homme - 50 % dosis letal
        para el hombre (LD_{50}) 350 rad

        Gastrointestinal death, which cannot be
        arrested even by bone marrow transplantation
        Gastrointestinaler Strahlentod, der auch durch
        Knochenmarktransplantation nicht aufzuhalten ist
        Mort intestinal ne pouvant être évitée même avec
        une greffe de moelle
        Muerte radioactiva gastrointestinal que no se puede
        detener incluso con trasplante de médula ósea   >10000 rad

3. Natural background radiation - Höhe der natürlichen
   Strahlenbelastung - Irradiation naturelle - Nivel de
   carga radioactiva ambiental

        Cosmic radiation at sea level - Höhenstrahlung in
        Meereshöhe - Rayonnement cosmique au niveau de la
        mer - Radiación cósmica al nivel del mar   2 µR/h

        Environmental radiation above sedimentary rocks,
        limestone and sand - Umgebungsstrahlung über Sediment-
        oder Kalkstein und Sand - Irradiation d'ambiance au
        dessus d'un terrain sédimentaire, de calcaire, et
        de sable - Radiación ambiental sobre piedra sedimen-
        taria o calcárea y arena   2-5 µR/h

        Same above volcanic rock - Desgl. über vulkanischem
        Gestein - Idem au-dessus de roches volcaniques -
        Idem sobre roca volcánica   10-25 µR/h

225

Zones with exceptionally high background radioactivity
Zonen mit besonders hohem Strahlenuntergrund
Zônes ayant une radioactivité specialement élevée
Zonas con radiación de fondo especialmente elevada 1)
(Neendakara/Kerala - Guarapari-Brasil)   < 300 μR/h
(Yearly doses - Jahresdosen - Doses annuelles -
Dosis anuales mR/a ≈ μR/h x 10)

4. Incorporated natural radionuclides - Inkorporierte
   natürliche Radionuklide - Radionucléides naturels
   incoporés - Radionúclidos naturales incoporados 1)

   ^{14}C (Whole body - Ganzkörper - Corps entier -
       Totalidad del cuerpo)   1.6 mrem/a

   ^{40}K (Whole body - Ganzkörper - Corps entier -
       Totalidad del cuerpo)   10-20 mrem/a

   ^{210}Po (Bone - Knochen - Os - Huesos)   14 mrem/a

   ^{222}Rn (Whole body - Ganzkörper - Corps entier -
       Totalidad del cuerpo)   2 mrem/a

   ^{222}Rn (Lungs - Lungen - Poumons - Pulmones)   150 mrem/a

   ^{226}Ra (Whole body - Ganzkörper - Corps entier -
       (Totalidad del cuerpo)   3-5 mrem/a

   ^{226}Ra (Bone - Knochen - Os - Huesos)   35 mrem/a

5. Levels of genetically significant doses from man made
   exposures - Genetisch signifikante Dosen aus künst-
   lichen Strahlenquellen - Dose génétique importante
   provenant des sources de rayonnement artificielles -
   Dosis geneticamente significantes a partir de fuentes
   des radiación artificiales 1)

       Fall out 1975   2-4 mrem/a

   Medicine - Medizin - Médecine - Medicina
   (Developed countries - Industrialisierte Länder -
   Pays développés - Paises desarrollados)

       Diagnostic radionuclides   30-50 mrad/a

       Radiation therapy   2-3 mrad/a

       Diagnostic isotopes   0.3-1 mrad/a

   Radioactivity in consumer goods - Radioaktivität
   in Verbrauchsgütern - Radioactivité dans les biens
   de consommation - Radioactividad en productos de
   consumo   < 1-2 mrad/a

   Nuclear power - Kernkraft - Centrales nucléaires -
   Potencia nuclear (1975)   < 1 mrad/a

   Idem expected - Erwartet - Idem, attendu -
   Predicción (2000)   1-3 mrad/a

   Average exposure of X-ray diagnosticians in Germany
   Mittlere Exposition von Röntgendiagnostikern in
   Deutschland - Irradiation moyenne des radiologistes
   en Allemagne - Exposición media de rayos X por médicos
   diagnósticos en Alemania   160 mrad/a

6. Radiation risk after whole-body irradiation with 1 rem
   Strahlenrisiko nach Ganzkörperbestrahlung mit 1 rem
   Risque dûe à l'irradiation du corps entier avec 1 rem
   Riesgo por exposición del cuerpo total de 1 rem

   Leukaemia   1:100 000

   Carcinogenesis   1: 10 000

7. Blackening of photographic emulsions - Schwärzung von
   fotografischen Emulsionen - Noircissement des émulsiones
   photographiques - Ennegrecimiento de emulsiones
   fotográficas

   See page - Siehe Seite - Voir page - Ver página 184

8. Dosis which can be detected by solid-state dosimeters
   Dosen, die mit Festkörperdosimetern festgestellt
   werden können - Doses pouvant être mesurées par des
   détecteurs à l'état solide - Dosis detectables con
   dosîmetros sólidos 2)

   Change of color - Verfärbung - Modification de
   la couleur - Cambio de color
                                                    1 kR-100 MR

   Photoluminescence (PLD)   10 mR-10 kR

   Thermoluminescence (TLD)   50 μR-1 MR

   Exo electron emission (EED)   10 μR-100 R

9. Polimerisation of plastics - Polimerisation von
   Kunststoffen - Polimérisation des plastiques -
   Polimerización de plásticos   100-1000 krad

10. Radiation resistance of building materials
    Strahlenfestigkeit von Baustoffen - Résistance
    à l'irradiation des matériaux de construction -
    Resistencia a la radiación de materiales

    Plastics - Kunststoffe - Plastiques - Plásticos 10^7-10^{10} rad

    Ceramics - Keramische Stoffe - Céramiques -
    Materiales cerámicos 10^{10}-10^{14} rad

    Metals - Metalle - Métaux - Metales 10^{15}-10^{20} rad

Lit.: 1. UNSCEAR: Report of the United Nations, Scientific Committee
         on the Effects of Atomic Radiation, Off. Rec. XXVII Session
         Suppl. No. 25 (A/8725), New York 1972
      2. UNSCEAR: Ionizing Radiation: Levels and Effects, Vol. I
         Levels, New York 1972
      3. BEIR-Report: The Effects on Populations of Exposure to Low
         Levels of Ionizing Radiation, Nat. Acad. of Sciences
      4. GROSSE-SCHULTE, M. in E. SCHRÜFER: Strahlung und Strahlen-
         meßtechnik in Kernkraftwerken, Berlin: Elitera 1974
      5. BECKER, K., SCHARMANN, A.: Einführung in die Festkörper-
         dosimetrie, 56, Thiemig: München 1975

10. Subject index

10. Sachverzeichnis

10. Index

Related Titles

J. Gershon-Cohen: **Atlas of Mammography**

W. Wenz: **Abdominal Angiography**

S. Wende, E. Zieler, N. Nakayama: **Celebral Magnification Angiography.**
Physical Basis and Clinical Results

S. Takahashi, S. Sakuma: **Magnification Radiography**

T. Nomura: **Atlas of Cerebral Angiography**

Angiography/Scintigraphy. Symposium of the European Association
of Radiology, Mainz, 1–3 October. 1970, Editor: L. Diethelm

Advances in Cerebral Angiography. Anatomy – Stereotaxy – Embolization –
Computerized Axial Tomography. INSERM-Symposium, Marseille,
May 13–16, 1975. Editor: G. Salamon

Encyclopedia of Medical Radiology/Handbuch der medizinischen Radiologie
In 19 volumes (approx. 52 subvolumes) with contributions in German and
English. Further information upon request

N. Hassani: **Ultrasonography of the Upper Abdomen**

W. A. McAlpine: **Heart and Coronary Arteries.** An Anatomical Atlas for Clinical
Diagnosis, Radiological Investigation, and Surgical Treatment

Radiological Exploration of the Ventricles and Subarachnoid Space.
By G. Ruggiero et al.

G. Salamon, Y. P. Huang: **Radiologic Anatomy of the Brain**

A. Wackenheim: **Roentgen Diagnosis of the Craniovertebral Region**

Biological Aspects of Radiation Protection. Proceedings of the International
Symposium, Kyoto, October 1969. Editors: T. Sugahara, O. Hug

Springer-Verlag Berlin Heidelberg New York

Related Titles

H. Dertinger, H. Jung: **Molecular Radiation Biology.** The Action of Ionizing
Radiation on Elementary Biological Objects (Heidelberg Science Library, Vol. 12)

Frontiers of Nuclear Medicine/Aktuelle Nuklearmedizin. Editor: W. Horst

W. A. Fuchs, J. W. Davidson, H. W. Fischer: **Lymphography in Cancer**
(Recent Results in Cancer Research, Vol. 23)

K. Kawai, H. Tanaka: **Differential Diagnosis of Gastric Diseases**

A. S. Takahashi: **An Atlas of Axial Transverse Tomography and its Clinical
Application**

A. Wackenheim, J. P. Braun: **Angiography of the Mesencephalon.** Normal and
Pathological Findings

Journals

Neuroradiology
Organ of the European Society of Neuroradiology

Pediatric Radiology

Radiation and Environmental Biophysics
Fundamentals and Applications

Biophysics of Structure and Mechanism

Medical Progress through Technology

Springer-Verlag Berlin Heidelberg New York